"Maintenance of healthy arteries requires excellent oral health. Dr. Ellie Phillips delivers an easily understood method for establishing and sustaining superb dental wellness. Anyone wishing to avoid a heart attack or stroke should read this outstanding book."

—Dr. Bradley F. Bale and Amy L. Doneen, M.S.N., A.R.N.P, medical directors of Heart Attack & Stroke Prevention Programs

"*Kiss Your Dentist Goodbye* will enlighten the public *and dental professionals* on the simple and mostly unknown ways of reducing decay and improving oral health. After reading this book you will be asking yourself why this important health information isn't making headlines. Well, it's about to!"

—Chris Kammer, DDS, founder, Masters of Progressive Dentistry; founding member, American Academy of Cosmetic Dentistry; dental expert for *USA Today, Reader's Digest,* and *FOX News*

"I initiated this hygiene program into my dental practice in May 2011. The results have been absolutely amazing, but this is only half the story! I brushed and flossed every day since 1966, getting perfect reports from my dentist. Then salivary testing showed my gums harbored bacteria that raised my chances of a heart attack or stroke by 15 times more than normal. Using the techniques in *Kiss Your Dentist Goodbye* for three months, these bacteria were reduced to insignificant levels. This book will not only save your teeth, it may just save your life. The information contained in this book is priceless!"

—Ron Phillips, DDS

"Thought provoking, to say the least, *Kiss Your Dentist Goodbye* encourages individuals to understand the caries disease process, question traditional beliefs, and take a proactive role to improve the strength and health of teeth in their care. On the quest for prevention, Dr. Phillips has mapped a new road for consideration and an easy-to-implement lifestyle change."

—Diane Brucato-Thomas, RDH, EF, BS, FADDH; ADHA-HuFriedy Master Clinician Award 2008; Sunstar/RDH Award of Distinction 2002; fellow in Periodontology, American Academy of Dental Hygiene

"Having been engaged in pharmaceutical development for over twenty years, I have become skeptical of so-called novel approaches to treating disease. However, the oral health care system described in Dr. Phillips' book, *Kiss Your Dentist Goodbye*, is based on sound physiology and biochemistry. Colleagues, family members, friends, and I have used Dr. Phillips' system for years and have all experienced significant and persistent clinical improvement."

—Michael A. Rudy, MD; president, Cytologics, Inc. (a pharmaceutical research and development company)

"Most people hate going to the dentist, but this book explains how an inexpensive, easy technique can reverse tooth problems. Those who follow Dr. Ellie's advice will be amazed at the results."

—Dr. Marlene Merritt, applied clinical nutritionist and doctor of oriental medicine

"Xylitol is awesome! I have been recommending xylitol to patients for years. My patients that have gone out and bought xylitol are really into it. It is the most practical way to eliminate decay and plaque, as well as helping problems with dry mouth."

—Connie Sidder, RDH; practicing dental hygienist for thirty years and frequent contributor to dental hygiene magazines

"Empower yourself! Dental decay is a disease YOU can do something about. This book tells you what, why, and how to do it. You can end dental damage and gum disease—even reverse early cavities in the comfort of your home."

—Nancy Kehr, director, National School of Dental Assisting; consultant in dental practice management, Nancy Kehr Consulting

"At a time of dental care transition, Ellie Phillips has written an exciting contribution to energize the public. It is bound to generate considerable debate, and discussion, with dental professionals, academicians, and recipients of that care. It gives the public more information and encourages personal oral health maintenance and prevention, all the while being down to earth. Bravo! Dr. Phillips embraces an accumulated forty years in multiple professional environments. She has refined her knowledge and presented it in a patient-oriented fashion for all socio-economic backgrounds. She is a pioneer practitioner. "

—James R. Delaney, DDS, FAAPD; chief of dentistry, Children's Hospital of Michigan

"What Doctor Ellie teaches in this book works exceptionally well. Patients now have a chance to avoid expensive dental treatments. Ethical and caring dentists will want to teach this information to their patients. As the tireless champion of preventive dental care, Ellie is ushering in very necessary and long overdue change. Everyone will benefit from reading this book . . ."

—David Snape, author of *What You Should Know about Gum Disease*

KISS YOUR DENTIST GOODBYE

A DO-IT-YOURSELF
MOUTH CARE SYSTEM
for HEALTHY, CLEAN
GUMS *and* TEETH

Ellie Phillips, DDS

RIVER GROVE
BOOKS
www.rivergrovebooks.com

This book is intended as a reference volume only, not as a medical manual. The information given here is designed to help you make informed decisions about your health. It is not intended as a substitute for any treatment that may have been prescribed by your doctor. If you suspect that you have a medical problem, you should seek competent medical help. You should not begin a new health regimen without first consulting a medical professional.

Published by River Grove Books
Austin, TX
www.rivergrovebooks.com

Distributed by River Grove Books

Design and composition by Greenleaf Book Group
Cover design by Greenleaf Book Group

Cataloging-in-Publication data is available.

Print ISBN: 978-1-63299-119-5

eBook ISBN: 978-1-60832-044-8

First Edition

Dedication

In March 2007, the American Academy of Pediatric Dentistry published a tragic story on its website. Eight-year-old Raven Blanco, from Chesapeake, Virginia, stopped breathing while receiving treatment at a pediatric dental office. Mild sedation had been used to calm the girl during the course of treatment, but at some point Raven became unresponsive. Her family watched as the dentist tried to save her. An ambulance arrived about seven minutes later, but the emergency medical crew could not revive Raven. Why she died is a mystery.

Before Raven went to sit in the dentist's chair, she gave her father a ring from her finger. She said, "Daddy, hold this until I get out."

"And I'm [still] holding it. I'm going to give it to her when I see her. I'm going to tell her, 'Raven, I held it for you,'" said her father.

This book is dedicated to Raven Blanco.

For more information on the Raven Maria Blanco Foundation, visit rmbfinc.org.

All truth passes through three stages: first it is ridiculed, second it is violently opposed, and third it is accepted as self-evident.

—Arthur Schopenhauer, nineteenth-century philosopher

I will prescribe a regimen for the good of my patients according to my ability and my judgment and never do harm to anyone. If I keep this oath faithfully, may I enjoy my life and practice my art, respected by all men and in all times; but if I swerve from it or violate it, may the reverse be my lot.

—The Hippocratic Oath

If I wish to compose or write or pray or preach well, I must be angry. Then all the blood in my veins is stirred and my understanding is sharpened.

—Martin Luther

CONTENTS

Foreword ix

Preface.. xiii

PART I: DENTISTRY'S BREAKING NEWS

Chapter 1: Dental Attitudes.................................... 3

Chapter 2: How It All Began................................. 19

Chapter 3: Setting the Stage.............................. 3 1

PART II: MOUTH ACIDITY

Chapter 4: Caries and Cavities............................ 4 1

Chapter 5: Mouth Chemistry................................. 5 3

PART III: GUM HEALTH

Chapter 6: Plaque 6 7

Chapter 7: Gum Disease 7 5

PART IV: MYTHS AND TRUTHS

Chapter 8: Fluoride... 8 7

Chapter 9: Sealants 1 0 7

Chapter 10: Whitening..................................... 1 1 3

PART V: THE GOOD NEWS

Chapter 11: Food for Teeth.................................129

Chapter 12: Xylitol..145

PART VI: A SYSTEM FOR HEALTHY TEETH

Chapter 13: The Complete Mouth Care System
for Adults.. 163

Chapter 14: The Complete Mouth Care System
for Children 187

Frequently Asked Questions.................. 201

Glossary... 205

Notes 209

About the Author................................. 229

Index 231

Foreword

The Oral-Systemic Health Connection

Today, a healthy mouth means more than flashing a row of pearly whites. We know that oral health is linked directly to general health, and no one should believe they have oral health simply because they "don't have cavities."

Oral health means working for the ultimate health of everything in the mouth—the teeth, gums, jawbone, tongue, saliva, and the skin inside the mouth. Saliva coats the surfaces in the mouth and maintains the strength of teeth and the health of soft surfaces. With a healthy, nutrient-rich saliva bathing teeth each day, you will not only have cleaner gums and teeth but also improved general health!

Think of saliva as water in a fish tank. Think of your teeth as stones in the fish tank. You could polish (and floss) the stones until they were perfectly clean, but if the water in the tank were dirty, the stones would immediately get dirty again as soon as you finished cleaning them. On the other hand, once the water is clean and remains clean, the stones will stop getting dirty. Oral health becomes sustainable once the "water" in your mouth is cleaned and healthy. This is where the use of xylitol becomes an almost miraculous way to clean saliva of harmful oral bacteria. Xylitol is a white, crystalline sweetener derived from xylose, a natural sugar found in plant and vegetable fibers.

Regular consumption of xylitol not only helps to remove harmful mouth bacteria and reduce plaque, but also appears to promote the formation of a healthy film called the pellicle, which protects tooth enamel. Today, large amounts of money fund studies on the relationship between saliva and the pellicle in a healthy mouth. Changes in the composition of saliva or mouth dryness can damage the pellicle. Abrasive toothpastes or harsh chemicals (in poorly formulated rinses) can remove this layer, resulting in tooth sensitivity and enamel weakness. As the public shops for oral care supplies, how do they decide what to use? Advice from health professionals may not always be objective and can be influenced by persuasive marketing. Ask me how I know!

Dr. Ellie Phillips brings common sense to the world of toothpaste and mouth rinsing. She has an unbiased and passionate interest in sustainable health outcomes. She has investigated and observed hundreds of patients, tracking outcomes as they used specific pastes and rinses. Once convinced that her system worked, she began her tireless mission to educate other health professionals and patients across the globe. The world must hear this information now, but unfortunately there are not enough voices proclaiming this news from the rooftops and out in the streets. Consider yourself very lucky that Ellie is!

Oral disease can be life-threatening, but new tests are helping health professionals evaluate their patients' mouths and eliminate dependence on visual observations. In her chapter about diagnosis of cavities, Ellie talks about the problem of knowing when a cavity needs filling, as well as the problem of over-diagnosis. Not every tooth with decay necessarily needs a filling, but patients are almost never given the choice to heal the decay. The usual action taken is to cut out the cavity and pack in a filling. The good news here is exactly what Bob Dylan was singing about years ago: the times, they are a changin'!

I believe the future role of a dentist will be to help patients enjoy whole-body health through oral health. My personal concern for many years has been that gum disease, hiding below the surface, can be overlooked by visual inspection. So it doesn't surprise me that 85 percent of American adults today have now, or have had, unhealthy mouths (according to the surgeon general) and that this impacts their general health in many ways. Before cardiac surgery, before a knee or hip replacement, or before having a baby, it is vital to consider oral health. Infection generates tissue inflammation, which can negatively impact outcomes at other body sites. Dental screening prior to medical procedures and dental care to reduce the risk of life-threatening disease will likely connect your physician and dentist in the future as they work together to help you live a longer, healthier life.

Fortunately, the composition of our "salivary soup" indicates when there are problems in our bodies or mouths. Salivary changes can tell us when periodontal disease or cavities are present. We know that acidity damages teeth, and measuring salivary acidity is a tool to help patients understand fluctuation in oral acidity. These measurements show how emotional stress and poor diet can translate to body and mouth acidity, and they reveal the negative impact these conditions can have on us.

Salivary testing is set to become a useful tool for improved oral cancer screening and will allow for the best treatment outcomes. And the use of saliva as a diagnostic fluid is not limited to oral disease. The composition of saliva is altered by changes in circulating blood, and these changes can alert health professionals to imbalances, especially prediabetic conditions. With such connection between our mouth and our body, it should not surprise you if your dentist becomes interested in recommending dietary changes, nutritional supplementation, treatments, and protocols to stabilize and improve your oral health to an ultimate level—not just to improve your smile, but to improve your life!

—Dr. Chris Kammer

* * *

Dr. Chris Kammer is president, founding member, and board member of the American Academy for Oral Systemic Health. AAOSH was created to bridge the gap between health professionals from all disciplines and develop communication about the oral-systemic connection for improvement in patient health. Visit www.AAOSH.com for more information.

Preface

The great thing in this world is not so much where we are but in what direction we are moving.

—Oliver Wendell Holmes

If you are confused about tooth care, you are not alone. People without cavities usually believe either that they were lucky to have been born with strong, healthy teeth or that sealants or fluoride helped them. People with fillings and dental problems normally believe they deserve them because they missed out on regular cleanings, or they used too little fluoride, or they did not floss enough. By the time you finish this book, you will see that these are not the reasons you have good or bad teeth. Dental problems can almost *always* be traced back to acidic or dry-mouth conditions, both of which encourage infection through harmful mouth bacteria.

Dentists have treated damaged teeth for decades with drilling, fillings, crowns, and powerful prescriptions. Any bad tooth part is cut away with a drill, and the cleaned tooth (or whatever remains of it) is rebuilt or covered. Dental repairs need maintenance, and because the disease that caused the problem was never cured, dental troubles usually persist. Traditional care may help you live without pain, but it does not stop the contagious bacterial infection that caused the damage in the first place. More and more dentists now realize this fact, and many have started to evaluate their patients' risk for dental disease, looking at all the possible reasons. This kind of dentistry is called *caries management by risk assessment*, and it is often combined with a conservative approach to fillings, where the least possible treatment is prescribed, called *minimally invasive dentistry.*

The truth has been known for years: Cavities and gum disease are preventable, and weak, damaged teeth can to some extent be naturally rebuilt and repaired *without* fillings. I encourage you to stop blaming yourself or your genes for dental problems. I will show you that dental disease is an infectious disease that you can easily control and stop. The system I recommend is radically different from the systems suggested by most dental offices, and using the system will give you radically different results.

I realize the high regard that many people have for the dental profession and the special affection patients often feel toward their dentist. My plan is not to end this relationship. Rather, I want to help you enjoy your teeth through a method that lets you achieve the ultimate dental health that both you and your dentist have been searching for. Once you are empowered by this simple system, you will most likely find that dental visits will become more rewarding and happier experiences, something you can look forward to without fear, emotion, or worry.

Imagine loving dental visits!

PART ONE

Dentistry's Breaking News

A man can succeed at almost anything for which he has unlimited enthusiasm.

—**Charles Schwab**

The doctor of the future will give no medication, but will interest his patients in the care of the human frame, diet, and in the cause and prevention of disease.

—**Thomas A. Edison**

CHAPTER ONE

Dental Attitudes

A number of years ago I attended a continuing education course whose featured speaker was a world-renowned cosmetic dentist. The dentist was extremely talented at fixing and re-creating natural-looking teeth. Instead of cutting down a tooth and sending an impression to a laboratory to make a cover or crown for it, this dentist left the original damaged or stained part in place and built a repair on top of it, directly in the mouth. Within an hour, he could mix porcelain-like pastes together and sculpture a new creation, adding shades of color to magically turn something broken and ugly into a perfect and natural-looking tooth.

The introduction to his course was a slide show of before and after pictures. We looked at patients old and young whose teeth were damaged, stained, and broken. Many of their teeth resembled little brown stumps in great need of a dramatic makeover. Cosmetic dentists from all over the world attended this course to learn about this particular repair method, materials, and techniques.

I raised my hand to ask a question. "Excuse me, but why do these patients have so much tooth damage?"

I felt the eyes of everyone in the audience stare at me in disbelief, as if I had asked the question in a foreign language. Why was I interrupting and wasting time? This was not the reason so many people had gathered together for the weekend. The dentist had no answer as to why his patients had so much erosion and damage to their teeth, so the lecture moved on.

In the years since then the speaker has become my friend. He has a great deal of interest in the prevention of dental disease, erosion, and tooth wear. In his office, patients are regularly interviewed to discover the cause of their dental damage and, even before his makeover treatments, they're counseled on how to prevent similar problems from occurring in the future. Today this dentist is a strong proponent of xylitol and the preventive program I recommend. He understands that although people come to him simply wanting good-looking white teeth, he needs to give them not only a beautiful new smile but also a way to keep it healthy and prevent future relapse. Without making some kind of change, the same problems that cause the initial tooth damage will cause the new "makeover" treatments to fail—often in less than three or four years.

Dentists and Prevention

Since ancient times, dentists have been viewed with trust and dignity. In Egyptian tombs, hieroglyphs have been uncovered showing an eye over a tusk. They date back to the fifth dynasty, indicating that even then, dentists were honored for their treatment of teeth. Today the profession continues to be made up of caring people who diligently follow the systems and teachings they learned at dental school. As their careers unfold, dentists expand their knowledge by attending seminars or courses and by reading books or professional journals.

The problem is that once a dentist graduates, he or she is usually too busy dealing with the daily workload of private practice to hunt for ideas that have not been presented at dental school, in journals, or during continuing education programs. In the United States, the majority of dentists have been trained to believe that prevention is flossing, diet control, regular dental cleanings, fluoride in the water, and oral examinations. Many dentists are unaware of other methods that effectively stop dental problems. Most believe it is impossible to halt dental disease.

In dental school, for example, we never discussed such variables as acidic saliva or mentioned tooth damage that occurs directly from acidic foods or drinks in the mouth. Not one of us ever thought to inquire whether foods or beverages like lemon juice or soda created acidic problems for teeth. We were never shown how to test the acidity of saliva or told about how it varies from person to person, from day to day, and even from situation to situation. Only one "fact" was hammered into our brains: Sugar causes cavities!

Dental training taught us to fear sugar and any food containing sugar or carbohydrates. Good dentists made patients worry about most of the foods in their home pantry: fruits (too many sugars); potatoes (too much starch); cereals, breads, potato chips, and crackers (too much of both); and of course candy, cookies, cakes, chocolates, and other desserts. Dr. R. M. Stephan's graphs from the 1940s alerted us to the danger of snacking: a colorful zigzag line that never reached a level of safety because there was no time for recovery between the "sugar attacks."[1] Few dental students have discussed food interactions, the benefits of tooth-protective ingredients in a meal, or how to reduce acidity with tooth-friendly foods.

The majority of dentists think that patients should control their sugar and starch intake and floss better if they wish to improve their

oral health. Unfortunately, you can diligently follow these procedures and still experience dental disease. Consequently, dentists have
become discouraged about prevention, and most are resigned to a
career of fixing their patients' ongoing dental problems.

A New Type of Dentistry

The knowledge of how to prevent cavities and gum disease dates back
to the 1960s, yet even today many people think it is difficult, perhaps
impossible, to have healthy teeth. Children and adults with bad teeth
often do not know the reasons for their problems. Too many people
subscribe to an antiquated notion that worn teeth, chipped enamel,
sensitivity, or bleeding gums are inevitable, or at the very least are a
part of the aging process. Some people blame their troubles on insufficient flossing or too few cleaning appointments. People are aghast if
I tell them it is possible to have strong, clean, bright teeth and healthy
gums *without* regular dental cleanings and even without flossing.

Dentists will always be necessary to fix broken teeth and make cosmetic changes to beautify a smile, but when you have finished this
book, you will understand why dentists cannot be the ones to prevent
your cavities or stop dental disease in your mouth. Weak, soft, or old
teeth are frequently given as excuses for dental problems, but these
descriptions do not explain *why* you have tooth damage. Finding out
why you have cavities or bad teeth is an important step toward preventing these problems and stopping the same damage from recur-
ring in the future.

Imagine that water is damaging a floor in your home. Before you
can fix your floor, you must find out where the water is coming from.
If you cannot find the cause, no matter how many floor repairs you
make, more water damage will occur. The only way to fix your problem is to find the source of the water, stop it, and then repair the damage. It is the same with your teeth. Where is the damage coming from?
Until you find the source of your tooth problems, repairs will need to

be done over and over, possibly getting more expensive and complicated each time. To put an end to soft, weak, stained, brittle, or sensitive teeth, you must first find out what is causing the damage.

Dentists have known for years that damaged enamel can be hardened back to total health with a simple repair process that occurs naturally in the mouth.[2] Under certain conditions, minerals from saliva can flow into teeth to strengthen them and in this way can even repair a cavity and prevent the need for a filling.[3] In 1999 a small group of dentists founded the World Congress of Minimally Invasive Dentistry to focus on prevention of dental disease and to promote techniques that preserve teeth and limit treatments that cut or damage them. These dentists believe in preventing dental disease by intercepting its progress with the least destruction of tooth tissue possible. Many of them recommend xylitol and explain natural tooth healing to their patients. In 2000 an international review paper described how dentists can use a natural repair system to limit the need for dental fillings and as a result practice minimally invasive or "minimal intervention" dentistry.[4]

A list of the world congress's members can be found at its website: www.wcmidentistry.com.[5] The Federation of Dentistry International also endorses a preventive approach to preserve teeth and allow natural healing to occur.[6] In addition, many pediatric dentists are familiar with a minimalist approach to treatment called *atraumatic restorative treatment.*

In the summer of 2006, the *New York State Dental Journal* published an editorial suggesting that dentists should educate patients about the "biological price" of dental treatment, particularly when other options, including an option of no treatment at all, exist. This was one of the first times I had seen anyone voice a concern about dental treatments and offer the idea that "no treatment" may be a benefit to the patient. Many dentists, like me, worry about the health impact of materials used for fillings, especially mercury-containing silver or white plastic compounds that may leach destructive ingredients.

Why place a filling if there are natural and possibly safer options? The respected author of the editorial appears to believe that there should be greater emphasis on communication in the dental office and that this exchange of information will, in the long run, help dentists retain public confidence.[7] I wholeheartedly agree with this concept and hope that dentists will promote more in-office dental conversations with patients about treatment choices for their dental health.

Today oral-care and dental-material companies orchestrate most American education programs for dentists. At a recent conference I was amazed to hear the worldwide director for one such company say that oral disease is not preventable. Her company educates dentists yet benefits from continued dental disease, so ask yourself: Would this be the most likely source for information about simple techniques that eradicate dental disease or for inexpensive, non-patentable methods that patients could use to maintain their own teeth in total dental health for life?

The subject of preventing dental disease has appeared to be absent from most major dental meetings, journals, and continuing education courses during the past twenty years. Since becoming a resident of the United States, I have searched for courses about mouth acidity, xylitol, or the process of natural tooth repair called *remineralization*. What I have found, instead, are courses on practice management, pharmacology, emergencies in the office, and many other sides of dentistry that fix and repair teeth. In 2001, however, I noticed that the National Institutes of Health, headquartered in Bethesda, Maryland, was looking at how dentists diagnose and manage dental disease and how to prevent cavities.[8] Naturally, I traveled to the meeting with excitement, and I was not disappointed, finding the information fascinating as well as helpful.

USING THE EXPLORER

One subject covered at that conference was the use of a device that dentists call an *explorer*. The sharp-pointed instrument has been a favorite dental tool for decades. The dentist holds the explorer in one hand and a small mouth-mirror in the other. Together, the explorer and the mirror allow the dentist to examine and feel the surface of your teeth, finding softened areas on their surfaces or any cavities or tooth decay that may have developed.

In the 1950s, it was common for dentists to force the instrument's sharp point against the surface of your tooth in their search for so-called sticky spots or potential cavities. Dental students were taught to push the point into any suspicious area and see if it could break the surface of the tooth, which would indicate this area needed a filling. By 1966, studies showed that softened areas on teeth could completely heal themselves with correct care, and that a cavity will disappear when minerals are replaced in it. Pushing a sharp point into a weakened area on a tooth reduced the chance of such a repair.[9]

Natural tooth enamel can rebuild itself and heal a soft spot, and this occurs quickly if the surface of the tooth remains intact. The repair process becomes more complicated and difficult, even impossible, however, if the surface is broken.[10] A study published in 1992 in the journal *Caries Research* reported on 100 teeth that had been examined with the explorer, been found to have sticky spots, and been extracted. The teeth were then cut into pieces and examined under a microscope to see whether the diagnosis of a cavity was accurate. Only 24 percent of the teeth with sticky spots had real disease and decay. The study showed how unreliable the explorer technique is for finding a cavity.[11]

Today any dentist who believes in natural repair of teeth would never forcibly push an explorer into a tooth surface. He or she would trail a blunted instrument over the tooth surfaces to check for roughened areas. If any were found, the dentist would suggest ways to harden and repair these soft spots naturally, remineralizing the softened areas until they went away and left a healthy and strong tooth.[12]

Obviously, pushing the explorer into the tooth can increase the chance of forming a cavity and may prevent a repair that otherwise would have been possible. The explorer can give a false reading, especially if the point is pushed into grooves on the biting surfaces of teeth. A few dentists remain determined to use the explorer in the time-honored way, claiming it is efficient standard care that is well accepted by the profession, insurance companies, and patients. There are dentists both for and against the "strong" use of an explorer on your teeth. Which kind of dental examination would you prefer?[13]

WHEN DOES A TOOTH NEED A FILLING?

Another subject for debate is *when* a tooth requires a filling. Until recently, it was your dentist's judgment call. Of course, if you have lost a chunk out of your tooth or if it is giving you pain, the decision may be obvious. The dilemma presents itself when the cavity is in its beginning stages,[14] a scenario that occurs regularly in dental offices every day in America.

One dentist may suggest a filling or a sealant to fix a tooth that has a softened or weakened area, usually visible on an X-ray. When a tooth with porosity or lost minerals or softened parts is X-rayed, the X-rays are able to travel through the empty or liquid-filled spaces more easily than through a harder, healthy tooth. X-rays of a hard or dense tooth bounce off the surface and make the image lighter or brighter in the film. The weakened tooth areas will be a dark or even black shadow against the brighter surface on the resulting film.

One dentist may see a shadow and suggest a filling. An equally qualified dentist may take a sequence of X-rays at regular intervals to see if the tooth is regaining its strength or weakening, explaining to the patient that he or she needs to go home and use a program that will strengthen and rebuild the softened tooth. The second dentist is giving the patient a chance to repair the softened area with natural healing so as to avoid a filling.

A weakened tooth can be rebuilt to total strength in a matter of months. With correct home rinsing and the use of xylitol (which are discussed in detail in chapters 13 and 14), a patient may be able to fix this kind of defect and never need a filling. If preventive treatments are not followed, however, the cavity could potentially become worse and spread into the live area deep inside the tooth. If that happens, the consequences would be more extensive treatment and possible damage to the central nerves of the tooth. Which decision is correct from an ethical standpoint?

Some dentists do not believe in natural tooth repairs because they have never seen a tooth rebuild itself. Without guidance, how would they become confident in the outcome? Dentists in a group practice may not see the same patient over time. An older dentist may have experience, but a young dentist may be solely dependent on his or her schooling. Consequently, the decision about whether to fill your tooth may be influenced by the age of your dentist, whether he or she has attended preventive lectures, or if he or she has interacted with other professionals knowledgeable about the natural rebuilding of teeth.

Perhaps your fillings could have been avoided. Research clearly shows disagreement among dentists about when a cavity requires a filling. A different study conducted in 1992 showed that the most likely error dentists make is filling a sound tooth, which happens when dentists look at X-rays and use traditional methods of diagnosis. They often decide to fill teeth that actually do not need filling.[15]

Fortunately, new technology is helping dentists make decisions more accurately, and with public demand, more people may be given preventive options.

WHAT TYPE OF FILLING SHOULD BE USED?

There are many good reasons to avoid fillings and to prevent gum disease at all costs. Over the past twenty years, a number of dentists have been so concerned about silver filling materials that they have removed them for the sake of their patients' health. Silver fillings are a mixture (an amalgamation) of metals that include almost 50 percent mercury. Mercury is a liquid metal used to bind the other dry metals together, just like an egg or oil is used in a cake mix. Like steam, however, mercury can vaporize and is toxic to humans when it is inhaled, ingested, or absorbed through the skin.

Today dentists no longer handle mercury or mix silver fillings directly. The ingredients are in capsules that are mixed automatically without contact with the skin. In many countries, organizations are trying to limit the use of mercury in health care and other industries.[16]

The argument in favor of silver fillings is that they have a long history in dentistry. The American Dental Association (ADA) claims that "the best and latest available scientific evidence indicates it [amalgam] is safe."[17] Records indicate that about 70,000 kilograms of mercury are used in more than 100 million dental fillings each year. Most dentists say they prefer amalgam over white filling materials for molar teeth.

Despite this endorsement, many people distrust silver fillings. In Sweden, Denmark, Germany, and Austria it is illegal to use silver fillings; a dentist can go to jail for using them.[18] It is now illegal in California to put silver fillings in the mouth of a pregnant woman because mercury can transport across the placenta and also enter mother's milk. In every dental office, old fillings or extra filling material must be placed in a special container and disposed of as toxic hazardous waste. If fillings break down in the mouth, it is easy for patients to eat or swallow pieces of them by mistake. Crumbling and failed fillings appear in acidic mouths, and some people have silver fillings replaced frequently throughout their lifetime, exposing themselves to mercury poisoning at each repair.

Statistics show that more than half the silver amalgam fillings put into teeth eventually need repair. The average life span of an amalgam was found to be 12.8 years, although that of a white filling was even less, only 7.8 years.[19] Consider a single tooth and how many times one filling may be repaired over a lifetime. Imagine if a filling is originally needed in a molar tooth at the age of five or six. How many fillings will four of these molars need throughout a person's life? Imagine a mouth full of fillings and the possible exposure to mercury these may cause. In an acidic, diseased mouth, fillings deteriorate quickly and may need replacement more often, even every few years, potentially exposing you to even more mercury and metal harm.

Drilling out old amalgam must be regarded as a serious procedure because high amounts of mercury vapor are released in the process. Extreme care should be taken to perform the procedure safely and with adequate protection, ideally with strong suction and a barrier to stop removed pieces or amalgam dust from being inhaled by the patient. The International Academy of Oral Medicine and Toxicology has established safety guidelines. Vapors from the new filling are equally problematic, and no excess filling should be left in the mouth in case it is accidentally ingested. These particles may be dangerous to health, especially for young or growing children. Your dentist should provide you with an alternative source of air during the procedure to keep you from inhaling mercury vapor.

If you prevent mouth acidity from damaging your silver fillings, they can last for decades, even for your whole life. As a geriatric dentist, I often saw fillings that had been placed in childhood still strong after sixty or more years. On the other hand, in an acidic and diseased mouth, fillings I personally placed with maximum care were leaking and failed within two years, not because of the materials but because of acid erosion around the filling, causing the enamel holding the filling to flake away.

If you have a healthy mouth, silver fillings can remain stable. Personally, I consider it safer to leave them in place rather than rushing to change them to another material. I would encourage everyone to protect and strengthen their enamel, because at this time there do not seem to be any perfect alternatives. Even white filling materials have safety questions, and few studies have been conducted to evaluate them. In addition, plaque bacteria appear to stick more readily to white fillings than to silver or gold ones. Gold or porcelain may be the best choice for molar teeth, but be aware that if gold and silver fillings are both present in an acidic mouth, they can mimic the chemistry of a battery and even create an electrical current.

Dental materials are changing all the time, so if you need a filling, discuss the topic with a trusted dentist and learn the advantages and disadvantages of the dental materials he or she suggests. The Internet is a good resource, but check the source of your information, and remember, the ADA has supported silver fillings since the 1800s. Ask about the safest filling materials and which ones are the most durable. If your dentist talks about watching a questionable tooth, remember how much healthier it is to have perfect teeth and find out if natural remineralization is an option.

New Techniques in Dentistry

Special equipment involving ultrasonic depth testing has recently been developed to help measure the strength of a tooth and display it in picture form on a computer screen.[20] It is now easier for a dentist to detect weakness in your tooth in time to warn you of an impending cavity. With that knowledge you could go home and rebuild your tooth using the repair process I describe in chapter 13. It is relatively easy to monitor the effects that products have on teeth because changes can be observed and measured. For example, if a product claims to strengthen or repair your teeth, you may notice the difference yourself, but we now have the technology to measure tooth strength and confirm if such claims are true. [21]

Today it is possible to take a digital picture or make a videotape of a tooth and view a cavity healing and shrinking in size. You can literally watch tooth damage disappear as minerals go into a tooth and repair it.[22] Your progress and improvement could be evaluated and measured at regular intervals with this kind of monitoring equipment.

To detect areas of softening not yet visible to the eye, special lights with attached computer systems have been developed. One method uses a Digital Imaging Fiber-Optic Trans-Illumination (www.difoti.com) and another, the DIAGNOdent laser, lights up bacteria by-products in a tooth (www.kavousa.com). There is also a fluorescent light, called the InspektorPro, which shows the relative strength of a tooth (www.omniipharma.com). The light causes a pattern that can be seen on a computer screen, with different colors corresponding to various degrees of tooth hardness.[23] This kind of light can therefore be used to show if, and by how much, a tooth has hardened up after a patient has used tooth-restoring measures. This method will eliminate the guesswork and help patients, and dentists, see that preventive treatments are working. If your dentist informs you that a tooth or teeth are starting to soften, you would then have time to prevent a cavity by using healing methods in a dental office or at home before the damage becomes irreversible. You should be visiting the dentist for a screening to help you prevent cavities rather than for treatments and fillings.[24]

Many people find this idea exciting, especially if the result is a lifetime of perfect teeth. Some dentists, on the other hand, do not think a cavity is a big deal; they may lack confidence in tooth repair and may have never seen a tooth rebuild itself. These dentists may worry that if a patient does not comply well enough, a small cavity could progress and become bigger. A home repair method depends on you, not the professional skill of the dentist. Such concerns may be reasons why dentists have ignored natural repair, choosing fillings instead. I believe that patients should be given the chance to choose between natural repair to heal a tooth and traditional repair with a filling.

Dentists as Evaluators and Fitness Trainers

Patients certainly expect dentists to be concerned about helping them avoid tooth loss and disease, but the role of dentistry in the future will be much more than this. The impact of bad oral health on general health has not been fully understood, nor the benefits of maintaining a healthy mouth. Blood chemistry is reflected in the quality of our saliva, and dentists should be monitoring this to alert patients of their general health. In a similar way, infection in the mouth will affect the outcome of surgery elsewhere in the body. Before any cardiac or replacement surgery, oral health should be examined in detail.

Patients should seek out dental professionals who believe in pre-vention and who will help them *avoid* treatments. I hope that dentists will be viewed more as dental evaluators who use their expertise to alert patients in advance of a cavity, so that patients can take steps to avoid the need for fillings or treatments.[25] You may have decided to select your current dentist because he or she accepts your insurance plan, but in the future you may think about selecting someone who believes in remineralizing teeth and who is known for a caring and effective approach to preventing dental disease.

Imagine if your dentist could alert you that your teeth were about to soften and give you time to prevent cavities in them with heal-ing home-treatment methods, before the need for fillings. If you kept regular visits they would be for screening and to help you prevent cavities so that you would never again need to go to the dentist for extractions, root canals, or fillings.[26] I believe the future of dentistry is a "drill-free" dental office.

Dentists who help their patients enjoy healthier teeth see posi-tive changes in their offices. Dentists who help patients take control of their dental health develop new relationships, especially as their patients become confident about dental visits. The number of broken appointments is reduced, and although less treatment may be done, more patients can be seen each day. Furthermore, happy patients refer many others.

The best news is how simple it is to prevent dental problems with correct home care. By using the system I describe in part VI, you will find that by yourself you can begin to successfully avoid cavities and many annoying dental problems. You can begin the preventive program whenever you choose, and because it is simple and convenient, you will most likely find that it quickly becomes an enjoyable and rewarding daily routine that you will use forever.

CHAPTER TWO

How It All Began

For millions of people, going to the dentist is a major source of stress and anxiety. Given the history of dentistry, and the fact that most people feel they have no control over dental problems, their fears are hardly a surprise. When I was growing up in England, it was not unusual to hear parents threaten to take a misbehaving child to the dentist *as punishment.* Those who have had negative dental experiences as children are often patients who experience the worst anxiety as adults. Ironically, in my case, the name of our school dentist was Dr. Dagger!

Early in My Career

Dental health for children was never a priority in England when I was growing up, and tooth extraction was considered a quick and easy solution for most dental problems. Things were actually so bad that dentures were given to some young people as wedding gifts, the idea being that extractions at an early age could ward off a lifetime of pain, problems, and expense.

My training as a dentist began at London University in the mid-1960s. I was fortunate to have been there then, as my teachers of dentistry at Guy's Hospital presented exciting new ways to protect and strengthen teeth. For the first time, the inevitability of tooth decay and tooth loss was being challenged. We were shown how, with correct care, patients could completely avoid the cavities and extractions previously believed to be a part of life.

We learned about the chemistry of the mouth and the biology of cavities and how dental problems could be prevented and even reversed. It was amazing to realize how easily patients could use a natural process to strengthen, protect, and even repair teeth on their own. The idea of a world where everyone could enjoy dental health without cavities or gum disease was very exciting.

My first job after dental school was working as a dentist in Lausanne, Switzerland. The Swiss dental insurance system appeared to favor healthy teeth and the prevention of dental problems. As the size of cavities and fillings increased, so did patient co-payments, providing a financial incentive for people to visit their dentists regularly, to learn to care for their teeth, and to keep cavities as small as possible. Patients used rinses and foods to strengthen their teeth and keep them healthy, thus avoiding fillings, crowns, and root canals. Extractions were rare, and dentures appeared to be regarded as a last resort when all other options failed.

I chose to start my career in Switzerland because I was concerned about the British National Dental Care System. Later I was excited to take the new techniques that I had experienced and use them to help improve treatment for patients in England. Dental health care in England at that time was driven by factors that did not seem to be in the patient's best interest. Under the government-operated system, dentists were paid on a sliding scale keyed to the size of a filling. The bigger the filling, the larger the fee. Money and ethics often clashed. Exaggerating the size of a filling could increase the dentist's income, and no one would be the wiser. "Extension for prevention" was a professional joke about making a filling bigger than it needed to be, leaving so little tooth, there was nothing left to decay. Dentists were well reimbursed for extractions, so they became the commonplace solution to dental problems. Some dentists had daily quotas to meet, and because the patients had no financial stake in the process, they quietly accepted the treatment. Extractions were common, as were overfilled, crowded, crooked, damaged, and stained teeth. The unfortunate system of dental care provided generations of comedy routines and jokes about ugly, unhealthy British teeth.

My first job in England was as a community dentist in a school clinic in the early 1970s. The clinic was a large room with one dental chair in the center. After greeting the office staff on my first day, I opened the door to welcome my first patient. A thirty-foot bench extended from the doorway to the end of the hall, and it was filled with at least twenty small children waiting to have their teeth extracted. Strained little faces looked at me with round, moist eyes. Mothers resigned to the inevitable sat beside their children with an air of compassionate authority.

That was the era when adults believed that children should be seen and not heard. Children were expected to sit quietly and handle whatever came their way. They were expected to undergo drillings or tooth extraction without complaining or crying—and, often, without an anesthetic. When the treatment was over, they were required to politely shake hands and thank the doctor and the office staff.

One by one the children silently came over to me. I was expected to extract their teeth according to the treatment plan I had been given. My head was spinning. I didn't know whether to carry out the dreadful treatment or to send them away. I did what I was expected to do, but I vowed from that day forward that by whatever means I could, I would help children everywhere enjoy healthy teeth and avoid cavities, fillings, and unnecessary extractions.

I began the next part of my career taking a closer look at the dental health of the children in my local community. I found an epidemic of tooth decay: babies with cavities and preschoolers with abscesses, lost teeth, and pain. I started a preventive dental program to teach pregnant women and young mothers how to look after their teeth and the teeth of their infants and toddlers. Because I was alone in the project, I divided the children into groups, sending older children with large cavities to family dentists who were happy to fill them with big and lucrative fillings. I used temporary fillings for baby teeth that were soon going to fall out, and I worked hard on behalf of the younger children, teaching their parents ways to prevent cavities.

I used permanent fillings in newer baby teeth instead of extracting them. Baby teeth are important because they hold a space for the permanent successor that grows between the roots, underneath in the jaw. Without baby teeth as placeholders, adult teeth can move around in the jaw, finally erupting out of line. Without a baby tooth, six-year molars can move forward and crowd out teeth that erupt in front of them a little later, during early teen years. Overcrowded teeth are difficult to clean and create traps for bacteria and plaque.

Baby teeth are also important as indicators and potential carriers of dental infection to newly erupting adult teeth. Children with cavities in their baby teeth are found to be at much greater risk for cavities in their permanent adult teeth. My experiences in Switzerland had taught me that ending meals with a tooth-protective food could make a huge difference to dental health and also how important nighttime oral care is for children and adults.

My new patients were happy to take the steps I suggested, and we quickly saw dramatic improvements. It was an exciting time for me as I realized how eager people were to avoid dental treatments and how interested they were in a new kind of treatment I called *preventive dentistry*.

Before long I was visited by a government representative who was upset about the reduced number of extractions at the clinic. Someone had noticed that temporary fillings were being put in teeth, and a staff member had complained that I was just talking with people. I had arrived at a career crossroads, and it was obviously time to leave the school clinic.

The next part of my dental career began when I opened my own practice just a few doors away from the government clinic. Parents arrived in large numbers, and although normal treatments allowed under the government system were without charge, my patients were willing to pay a small fee to bring their children for this preventive program. I was different from most dentists in town; dental visits were no longer a cause of fear or terror for the children. I was a teacher and a coach. Furthermore, at that time a female dentist in a pantsuit was something of a British novelty.

As the years passed, the volume of patients I treated outgrew my office space to the point where I could not fit another patient in the door. Every day we were busy from early until late. On Saturday mornings we helped nervous children become familiar with the dental office by having them watch movies in the waiting room and play with the dental chair. Parents came to learn about taking care of their children's teeth, and the positive results soon became obvious to them.

The children were not developing cavities because they were following the simple procedures and preventive routines I prescribed. Mothers came in to take advantage of the new dentistry for themselves, followed by their sisters, mothers, husbands, fathers, aunts, cousins, and more. Whole families were learning and using my routines and techniques to prevent cavities and enjoy healthy teeth.

My office grew, and I saw more and more people with special needs who required sophisticated dentistry to save their damaged teeth. London was home to the Eastman Academy of Dentistry, and I took classes there to learn about treatments to care for the developmentally disabled.

The Eastman Dental Center

Some years later I moved to New York and worked with special-needs children in the Rochester area. I trained at the Eastman Dental Center in its residency programs for adult and children's dentistry. The Eastman Dental Center, long a sister establishment to London's Eastman Academy, is associated today with the University of Rochester. Ultimately, I became a member of the faculty at the University of Rochester and director of the Eastman Pediatric Outpatient Clinic.

The Eastman Dental Center provides graduate training for dentists in many specialties. The center was originally the vision of George Eastman, the wealthy philanthropist and founder of the photographic company Kodak. In 1917, Eastman donated part of his fortune to develop a system he hoped would prevent dental disease among the children of Rochester. Before that time, dental care was available only for the wealthy, and preventive dental care was unknown.

Many forward-thinking doctors at that time were connecting general health with nutrition. George Eastman believed in good nutrition and also that dental health and general health were closely aligned. When Eastman established his dental clinics, he hoped to start a movement that would improve the general and dental health of children all around the world. During the 1920s, Eastman organized training for groups of women who were called *prophylactic squads*, the pioneers in what became modern dental hygienics. The squads were sent to Rochester schools with dental chairs, instruments, and slides to teach toothbrushing. It was Eastman's hope that the children of Rochester would be the first of a future generation who would enjoy better teeth and less dental pain.

In London in the 1960s, the science of preventive dentistry was new and exciting. Thirty years later in the United States, I saw firsthand the painful reality of poor dental health almost a century after George Eastman established his dream, and I was appalled by the state of many children's teeth. To this day the children of Rochester continue to suffer fillings, abscesses, and extractions; many need sedation or a general anesthetic for dental work that is so lengthy and complicated it has to be done under surgical operating conditions. The majority of children seen at the clinic are preschool age, which makes the situation even more distressing.[1] Sadly, many of the children treated in the clinic have social and emotional challenges often made worse by their dental problems—problems that are preventable. As these children age, almost none will enjoy optimal dental health.[2]

Oral Health in America

Despite all the time and money spent, insurance coverage, and dental visits, one out of five Americans rates his or her oral health as fair to poor. Statistics show that almost a quarter of young people today between the ages of eighteen and thirty-four have gum disease and say their teeth hurt when they drink hot or cold beverages.[3] Rarely do any middle-aged or elderly people have white or perfect teeth. Dental problems are not about concern or time. Such problems exist because the majority of people do not know how to protect their teeth and keep them strong, attractive, and healthy. People assume that teeth crumble and wear out with age, and that gum disease is unavoidable.

In May 2000, U.S. Surgeon General David Stacher released a report about the status of oral health in America.[4] It was a report similar to the one Luther Terry had issued in 1964 about the relationship between tobacco and health. Both reports were designed to develop science and research on vital public health issues and were supposed to encourage, motivate, and mobilize the public to deal with serious health problems more effectively. Stacher's report included a call to action to improve an unhealthy dental situation across America. The situation was deemed especially serious for disadvantaged and minority children, who were found to be at the greatest risk for severe medical complications from dental disease.

In April 2003, Surgeon General Richard H. Carmona created a document called the "National Call to Action," which described the epidemic of dental disease sweeping through urban and rural districts of America.[5] Carmona talked of the need to build a science base for three purposes: (1) to examine treatment effectiveness; (2) to encourage dentists to make informed decisions; and (3) to accelerate public awareness. Even today, among educated circles in the dental profession, there remains a serious gap in basic knowledge about evidence-based effective ways to control and prevent dental disease.[6] Most disturbing is the lack of public awareness about methods that anyone could use to avoid dental problems.

Statistics from Carmona's report show that tooth decay is the single most common chronic childhood disease, five times more common than asthma and seven times more common than hay fever. The report further describes the impact that dental disease has on productivity among schoolchildren and employed adults. More than 51 million school hours are lost each year from dental-related illness; more than 164 million work hours are lost annually from dental disease or dental visits. The Department of Health and Human Services' Centers for Medicare and Medicaid Services estimated that the nation's total bill for dental services was $70 billion in 2002. With such horrible statistics, the questions must once again be asked: Why is there so much dental disease? Why have all the generally accepted methods of prevention been unable to stop it? What are the best ways for the public to avoid being a part of this problem?

Many city, rural, and suburban children in the United States need extensive fillings or extractions by kindergarten age. Statistics show that tooth decay in baby teeth is not declining, despite all the measures tried over the past forty years. More than half of first-grade children have cavities in their teeth; these are often in new adult molars. More than three-quarters of high school seniors have cavities, damage, or scarring on their teeth, especially around braces.[7]

An alarming number of teenagers are diagnosed with gum disease that may cause permanent damage to their teeth before they are twenty. Most of these children have seen dentists during their childhood, have been involved in school dental programs, and have been given regular cleanings, X-rays, and fluoride treatments. Ever-increasing amounts of Medicaid money have been spent, state-of-the-art clinics have been built, school-centered mobile units have been purchased and equipped, even high-tech teledentistry has been used to examine children, yet the problems continue to escalate. How can it be that with so much care, so many children have so much dental damage?

More people than ever seem to be experiencing brittle, weak enamel and sensitive teeth. Are oral care products or the overuse of corrosive, abrasive, or whitening products damaging dental enamel? Or is the decline of dental health related to modern American beverage consumption, medication side effects, stress, allergies, or the use of sugarless products that could promote acid reflux symptoms? Today most medications have mouth-drying side effects, and a dry mouth is a risk factor for dental problems (see chapter 4). The saliva that protects teeth also protects your esophagus. If the coating is absent from your teeth, it may also leave your esophagus vulnerable to bacterial or fungal infections that create symptoms of acid reflux (see chapter 5).[8] It is interesting how dry mouth, dental problems, and acid reflux are so closely linked.

A few years ago I visited a graduate dental program and talked with senior residents, some of the best dentists in the world. I asked if they believed dental disease was a preventable condition. The young professionals expressed pessimistic views about their patients' ability to floss. In the opinion of these senior residents, dental disease was solely the result of inadequate flossing. They seemed resigned to providing fillings, crowns, bridges, and other work to repair the inevitable damage they expected. It was obvious that these dentists viewed their responsibility as one of fixing dental damage to the best of their ability. Even before they entered the work world, the young dentists were blaming patients and had no confidence in any preventive process to stop fillings or other dental problems. They believed that, eventually, everyone needs some kind of treatment.

Despite this pessimistic outlook, not one of these dentists questioned whether flossing was a good preventive method or if there might be a better way to care for teeth that had been overlooked. Any dentist will confirm that for someone to question flossing, fluoride, or any other accepted treatment is professionally challenging, and those who have asked such questions have received hate mail, complaints from their peers, and worse.

Interestingly, there are no randomized clinical trials to show that flossing prevents cavities, yet dentists have collectively repeated the flossing mantra for fifty years. In the world of dentistry it is politically incorrect to question the usefulness of flossing. This would not be a concern if the outcome of this traditional dental advice had guided the population to a lifetime of healthy, white teeth. The problem is that in the USA today, almost 100 percent of adults—even those who floss regularly—eventually will succumb to and suffer from dental disease. Despite expensive treatments, flossing, dental cleanings, and regular dental visits, everyone is expected to end up with tooth loss and the need for artificial replacements.

Dentists Are Frustrated Too

You may be surprised to learn that even dentists and dental hygienists are usually pessimistic when you talk to them about dental health. They frequently express frustration with the ineffectiveness of patients' flossing and the outcomes they see in their patients' mouths. The problem is that too few professionals know of any alternative treatments to recommend. Most dentists willingly admit that they view their job as providing treatment to fix the damage that dental disease causes. They will tell you that the damage is the result of an uncontrollable, progressive disease that gets worse as people age.

Surely it makes sense to review the methods routinely prescribed and to look closely at research and studies that support new and effective alternatives.

I have always found patients very interested in advice about dental care. People of all ages want to improve the condition of their teeth as long as the suggestions are easy to use and fit the individual's lifestyle. What is the point of suggesting chewing gum to someone who does not chew gum? When dentists tell patients to floss more often, they forget that for many people flossing is difficult, annoying, or too time-consuming. People need to be enthusiastic about their tooth care routines, and most of all, people want to see positive results. Any system should be simple, tailored to the individual, and effective. It is easy to become discouraged if you have been told to give up your favorite food or use bad-tasting or expensive products (goop in trays, gels, and tasteless foams) that give poor results and that allow your dental problems to continue. With the program I recommend, you can enjoy your normal routines and eat and drink all your favorite foods and beverages, yet you will protect your teeth and achieve dramatically improved dental health.

CHAPTER THREE

Setting the Stage

Surprising as it may seem, many people are unaware that dental disease is just like any other infection caused by bacteria. It is a disease that can spread easily, is transferred from person to person, and worst of all, can grow on things like toothbrushes. Once you realize that dental disease is this kind of infection, you understand how very simple steps can be used to control it.

In the nineteenth century, progressive medical surgeons begged peers to wash their hands so as to prevent the spread of infection. Today I beg patients to clean their mouths and their toothbrushes to control the spread of tooth and gum disease between family members. Today we have become more aware of the delicate balance that exists between the bacteria that help and protect us and the bacteria that cause infection. Overuse of antibiotics showed us that if protective bacteria were removed, overgrowth by harmful ones often followed, and the same reactions can be seen when we look at mouth bacteria.

Bacteria

Bacteria that live on teeth can grow only when attached to a hard, non-shedding surface. Some kinds of tooth bacteria are harmful, whereas others are good for our dental health. In fact, it appears that teeth need a barrier of healthy protective bacteria to stop harmful ones from damaging the tooth surface. The balance between good and bad bacteria is important for dental health, and it is also important to know that this balance can change. People are often surprised to learn that they can lose healthy bacteria following an abrasive dental cleaning, after taking a course of antibiotics, or when the mouth becomes dry or acidic for long periods of time. During times of change, it is possible for a new type of bacteria to infect your mouth and suddenly cause damage to your teeth and dental health.

BACTERIAL TRANSFER

Tooth bacteria rarely exist in a baby's mouth before the presence of a tooth. Therefore, the origin of these bacteria is necessarily someone else's tooth. DNA studies have illustrated that a parent, usually the mother, is most often the person who passes tooth bacteria from her mouth to the baby's mouth when his or her first tooth erupts.[1] Most people imagine a genetic link or something in mother's milk that passes on dental disease. The truth is that dental disease is transferred directly to a child's new tooth, often during a loving cuddle or a kiss.

Most often, parents and caregivers share their mouth germs with their children (vertical transmission),[2] but it is also possible for mouth germs to spread between siblings or from spouse to spouse (horizontal transmission).[3] Parents should also be aware that children born by caesarean section appear to be infected by mouth germs earlier—possibly because they lack some kind of protection—than do vaginally delivered infants.[4]

Bacteria travel to the new baby tooth most often in a droplet of saliva. The bacteria can transfer during a kiss, from a drop of saliva on spoons or pacifiers, or from food shared with a baby. I would never suggest that parents stop kissing their baby or worry about sharing food. Think about this: If the bacteria do not come from your mouth, they will be transferred from the mouth of someone else who comes into contact with your child. Since this bacteria transfer cannot be stopped, it makes more sense to control the *kind* of bacteria passed to children.

Obviously, you want a baby to be infected with healthy, dentally protective bacteria rather than aggressive, cavity-forming ones.[5] The fact is that once a particular kind of bacteria reaches a baby's first tooth, this bacteria will then colonize or spread to the other baby teeth as they erupt. It has also been shown that whenever there are many harmful bacteria in a parent's mouth, the chances that they will transfer to the child are greater.[6] It has also been shown that the first kind of bacteria to infect the biting surfaces of molar teeth usually become the dominant strain in the mouth, because the grooves of these teeth become reservoirs of bacteria for the mouth. Changing the kind of bacteria in a child's mouth after molar teeth have erupted becomes more difficult. This fact can also be used to a parent's advantage—as you will see later on. To give children the best advantage, make sure that healthy bacteria are established in their mouths before the molar teeth erupt. This simple change can provide your child with many years of dental protection.

Research during the 1980s illustrated how bacteria were transferred between family members and from mouth to mouth. A simple and successful method of controlling this transmission was found just a few years later. For twenty years we have known how to reduce both the inheritance of bad tooth bacteria and the chance of a parent infecting their child with the bacteria that cause cavities. Parents with bad teeth can get rid of aggressive and harmful bacteria from their mouths, and even without traditional dental treatment. You may be shocked to discover that it is possible to remove harmful bacteria even if you still have cavities or cannot go to the dentist, for whatever reason. When the bad bacteria are gone from your mouth, protective ones will take their place.[7]

From a parent's point of view, it is important to know that the earlier a child is infected with harmful mouth bacteria, the greater the child's risk for having cavities later in life. As mentioned earlier, changing the kind of bacteria in your mouth becomes more difficult when molar grooves have become reservoirs of mouth bacteria.[8] Baby molar teeth erupt during the second year of life. Consistent with this fact are the results of studies showing that children who are infected with harmful bacteria by age two have the most cavities at age four.[9] When parents have healthy mouths during the first year of their baby's life, their children will have less chance of infection from harmful bacteria and a better chance for oral health. Studies have also shown that at five years of age, children from parents with healthy mouths have 70 to 80 percent less chance of developing cavities, and the benefits may last into adulthood.[10]

Preventing the passage of harmful germs to the next generation may be the most promising method of preventing cavities in children's teeth. If this is the first time you have heard about this kind of bacterial transfer, it will be natural for you to wonder why there has been no media attention and no national education on the topic.

For many years, dental associations in Europe and Scandinavia have been promoting such control of infant mouth bacteria as a means of improving oral health. Recently, a few state health organizations in the United States have begun to educate health professionals about oral bacteria transmission. Unfortunately, some of their recommendations seem unrealistic.

In 2007, for instance, the New York State Department of Health published a guide for oral care during pregnancy and early childhood.[11] The department's advice for preventing harmful bacterial contamination between mothers and infants and between siblings is that families should avoid saliva-sharing activities. Basically, they recommend that a mother not kiss her baby and that children not be allowed to share their toys. As a mother of five, I look at these recommendations and shake my head, wondering how anyone could even think of suggesting that a mother not kiss or share meals with her baby, or how anyone could recommend that toddlers not be allowed to play with one another's toys.

Even if a mother avoids kissing her baby, inevitably someone else will infect the child. Most parents would prefer to take ownership of this duty and prepare to pass healthy bacteria from their own mouths to their child. In daycare centers there are risks of contamination among children and also from caretakers. A study from a daycare center in Brazil suggests that horizontal transmission occurred among children in such situations.[12] Parents should understand these risks if their infant is in daycare and take some simple steps (as outlined in chapter 14) to keep their baby's teeth healthy and safe.

Mouth Chemistry

Mouth chemistry is affected by hormonal factors, poor diet, dehydration, and medications, especially those that change hormone levels, affect diuretic or liquid balance, or have the side effect of dry mouth. Sometimes changes in saliva flow and mouth chemistry occur so slowly that you can be unaware of your increased risk for cavities until problems arise.

Women's mouth chemistry in particular is volatile, and changes that make the mouth more acidic will have devastating effects on their teeth. A number of life situations can influence and cause the chemistry of the mouth to deteriorate. For example, new mothers who have enjoyed perfect teeth all their lives may be shocked to find cavities develop during their pregnancy. Sometimes the damage is seen as loose fillings, bleeding gums, or sensitive teeth. Hormones trigger a change in a pregnant woman's saliva, altering its quality and limiting its ability to provide natural tooth protection. These changes can occur at any time during a pregnancy, but the most risk for acidic damage to teeth occurs during the last trimester. (See chapter 13 for more details about changes in a woman's mouth chemistry during pregnancy.)

Other situations, many beyond your control, can suddenly increase your risk of dental damage without warning. One of the best ways to minimize the chance of cavities is to strengthen your teeth in advance of any problems and to protect teeth daily as much as possible. The following is a list of circumstances that can change your mouth chemistry by making saliva more acidic or by drying the mouth and, consequently, elevating the risk of developing cavities and other dental problems:

- Nasal congestion from seasonal allergies, asthma, or sinus infections
- Hormonal changes (including pregnancy, adolescence, and menopause)
- Medications (including Ritalin)
- Illness with fever or nasal congestion (even a simple cold or the flu)
- Mouth breathing (athletics, wearing dental braces)
- A chronic or acutely stressful situation, such as a death or crisis in the family, or business stress
- Duties that involve constant talking, such as lecturing, teaching, or stage performance
- Gastric acid reflux

- Bulimia
- Chemotherapy or long-term illness
- Poor diet, with lack of minerals and vitamins
- Fear
- Depression
- Dehydration
- Aging
- Work in situations where oxygen changes (divers, astronauts)
- A feeding or breathing tube in hospitalized patients

The idea of controlling mouth acidity may sound daunting at this time, but you will soon discover how simple routines can give teeth the protection necessary for dental health. Balancing mouth chemistry is relatively easy and will help you avoid dental problems.

PART TWO

Mouth Acidity

Let nothing which can be treated by diet be treated by other means.

—**Maimonides**

CHAPTER FOUR

Caries and Cavities

Many people believe that sugar is the main cause of cavities. They are unnerved when I explain the shocking myth buster: Sugar itself does not harm teeth. It is helpful to understand exactly how tooth decay happens; then you will see how easy it is to control. Teeth are damaged only when sugar energizes a damaging kind of bacteria in your mouth. Sugar gives energy to this particular kind of bacteria and they, in turn, produce tooth-corrosive acids. Acids weaken teeth and cause cavities. Let me restate this simply: Without the harmful acid-producing bacteria, sugar will not harm your teeth.

The interaction between bacteria and sugar was discovered and explored during the 1950s and 1960s. Testing was done on germ-free rats raised in a laboratory. The animals were bred without bacteria in their mouths, and although they were fed sugar and water for long periods of time, not one of them developed cavities. Different types of bacteria were introduced into each rat's mouth, and dental changes began to occur. Researchers found that one kind of bacteria in particular caused the most cavities to form in the animals. An antibiotic was used to eradicate these bacteria, and the tooth decay stopped. In other words, it was only when the specific bacteria were present in the animals' mouths that cavities formed.[1]

These experiments showed how mouth bacteria can use sugar from the diet to multiply, produce acidic liquids, and damage teeth. They also showed how the bacteria were transferred from mothers to their pups. Some bacteria were found to be more aggressive than others and produced more corrosive acids, causing the most cavities in teeth.[2] The damage we believed was from sugar was really damage from harmful mouth bacteria *fed* by sugar.

Whenever harmful mouth bacteria are energized and multiply, they damage tooth surfaces that are underneath or alongside them. The greatest damage will always occur where there is the most acidity. This is usually on the tooth surface in contact with the bacteria. When harmful bacteria continue to produce acids, over time these acids mix with saliva in the mouth and weaken teeth everywhere, even at a distance from the bacteria. Generalized mouth acidity is particularly dangerous because it encourages the growth of more acid-loving bacteria and the progression of this destructive, cavity-forming disease we know as tooth decay.

The 1960s studies illustrated the interaction between bacteria and sugar, yet even today most dentists and hygienists learn about sugar damage from the Vipeholm study, undertaken twenty years earlier. For decades dental students have been shown graphs that depict the results of this study, drawn by Dr. R. M. Stephan and carried out in a home for psychiatric patients in Sweden.[3]

The patients in this Vipeholm study lived in closed community conditions where harmful mouth bacteria would certainly have been present, and as a result, the bacteria of dental disease would have spread easily among them. These patients were obviously at high risk for dental disease. Their mouths would have been full of aggressive, acid-producing bacteria. We now understand how aggressive bacteria produce acids every time sugar is eaten. Something that is rarely explained to students is that in a mouth *without* harmful bacteria, acidity will not be produced and sugar will not harm teeth.

In the Vipeholm study, sugar was given to the residents and mouth acidity measurements were taken and related to measurements of tooth damage. Graphs were used to explain how sugar causes an acidic drop in the mouth and how this results in damaged teeth.[4] Stephan's diagrams are still used to illustrate how eating sugar makes the mouth acidic, too acidic for tooth safety. These diagrams are also used to show the time it takes for the dangerous acids to be diluted by saliva and for the mouth to return to a safe state. While the mouth is acidic, teeth are being damaged and cavities are developing.

Stephan's diagrams show that it takes about thirty minutes for saliva to balance the acidity and return the mouth to a safe state for teeth.[5] What is rarely explained is that this kind of balancing can occur only in a mouth with plenty of healthy nonacidic saliva. Obviously this balance cannot occur in a dry mouth without saliva or in a mouth where the saliva itself is acidic. This fact alone makes mouth acidity of extreme importance to everyone, especially for women in situations of hormonal imbalance, people who are taking medications, or people living under stress.

Dental Caries

People often think that dental caries is the same thing as cavities. A cavity is just a hole caused by *caries,* the disease that damages teeth. Many people think that cavities happen for no real reason, in any random place on a tooth, but cavities are not random at all; they are the result of damage caused by a bacterial disease that can easily be present on your teeth and all over your mouth. The infection of dental disease—that is, dental caries—will never be isolated to one place or one tooth; it attacks and weakens all your teeth at the same time. Once in your mouth, caries softens your teeth progressively until they break, usually one or two at a time, always at the most vulnerable places. When you understand these facts, you see why placing a filling in a cavity does nothing to stop the disease that caused it or the damage that this disease will now inflict on other teeth elsewhere in your mouth.

Dental caries can spread and become more damaging if particular factors, which I call *perfect storm conditions*, occur in someone's mouth. Mouth conditions deteriorate as harmful bacteria feed on sugars or starches in the diet. Sugars and starches supply these bacteria with energy that allows them to multiply and produce acids, which can make the whole mouth progressively more acidic. The acidity attacks and weakens tooth enamel everywhere, but the tooth enamel that is under the most stress from biting or chewing will usually be the first place to break and form cavities in teeth.

If conditions in your mouth do not change, one cavity will soon be followed by another one. If you do not eliminate the disease that caused the first problem, more damage will occur to other teeth, and you will most likely start a never-ending series of treatments. Over time, in an unhealthy mouth, the ongoing disease attacks the new fillings. Consequently, fillings fail and need repairs, then bigger fillings and eventually root-canal treatments and crowns. In a diseased mouth, most newly filled teeth show signs of damage and need repair within five years after the original treatment. In some cases it can be less time before a new filling needs repair.

INSIDE A TOOTH

Some people are surprised to learn that inside the outer shell of a tooth is soft living tissue with cells, nerves, and a blood supply. The outside of a tooth may feel hard to your tongue, but don't imagine your teeth as a row of stony pebbles in your mouth. If they were, it would be fine to scrub, bleach, and polish them because then, the more you scrubbed and polished, the brighter they would be. The fact is that the outer enamel of a tooth is a delicate mesh of minerals that is easily rubbed away, dissolved, and damaged, particularly by acidity or inappropriate scrubbing and polishing.

OUTSIDE A TOOTH

Weakness in the outer layer of your tooth can allow liquids, bacteria, and stains to travel toward the center part, which will irritate the nerve and potentially lead to an infection that can threaten the life of your tooth. Protecting tooth enamel is important for many reasons, but especially in order to keep the center of your tooth healthy and disease free.

The enamel on the outside of your tooth is constantly changing in strength and hardness, becoming softer for a while and then naturally hardening up again. People have known for years that there is a similar chemistry to keep our skeleton healthy. Minerals are deposited into bones and then removed in a natural process of breakdown and rebuilding. Healthy bone exists when the repairs balance the wearing away. Even under normal, healthy conditions, the strength of tooth enamel is always in balance, as the outer enamel builds up and breaks down all day and all night.[6]

Strong Teeth

As we grow older, or if sickness changes our body chemistry, repairs to our skeleton may slow down, and osteoporosis (thinning of the bones) can occur if there is not enough building up of bones to counter the wearing away. Changes in the balance make it difficult to maintain bone strength, and the same goes for teeth. For bone health, women are encouraged to build the strength of their bones before they become weak or damaged. They should similarly work to protect and maintain the strength of their teeth, even before they see any signs of damage.

The difference between maintaining healthy bones and teeth is the ease with which we can control the balance for our teeth and prevent any loss of strength in the enamel, no matter our age or our state of general health. Our teeth are in direct contact with mouth liquids that can either soften and wear teeth away or build them up. Everything we consume touches our teeth directly or mixes with mouth liquids to flow around them, into every groove or pit on their surface. Food particles dissolved in mouth liquids contribute either to tooth erosion or tooth repair, depending on the chemistry of the resulting liquid. When any corrosive or acidic mouth liquid flows over teeth, it interacts with the surface of the enamel and dissolves it.

MINERALS

If you examined healthy enamel with a microscope, you would see that it is made up of a skeleton with crystals in between a lattice-shaped structure. These crystals are packed tightly together, with only a very thin, watery film between them. Even when enamel is healthy and made up of these densely packed crystals, mouth liquids can flow between them, working through the tiny spaces around each crystal.

Tooth enamel is built from calcium and phosphate, two minerals that occur naturally in saliva. Under the correct conditions, these minerals combine to form crystals called *calcium hydroxyapatite*. These crystals are packed together tightly, like little grains of salt, within a lattice-type skeleton that creates the structure of tooth enamel. The appearance of enamel is like a honeycomb, and you can imagine the skeleton as the comb and the crystals like the honey that fills in the spaces.

When your saliva is alkaline, calcium and phosphate flow into tooth enamel and build more crystals that form strong and dense enamel that is resistant to damage. As you will see in chapter 5, on mouth acidity, in a moist and alkaline mouth, enamel crystals grow large and thick because minerals are plentiful. Most people are aware that fluoride helps to strengthen teeth and fluoride works by encouraging the formation of these large and well-formed enamel crystals.

In a moist and alkaline mouth, dilute concentrations of fluoride can increase the speed at which minerals from saliva turn into enamel crystals. Fluoride is really an activator—in scientific terms, fluoride would be called a *catalyst*. The interesting thing is that when enamel crystals form in the presence of fluoride, a tiny particle of fluoride is incorporated into the crystals. The scientific name of this crystal is calcium fluorapatite, and it has a different chemistry from the calcium hydroxyapatite crystal of regular enamel. Calcium fluorapatite is larger than regular enamel crystals and has a more perfect shape. Tooth enamel formed with this kind of crystal appears smoother, shinier, and stronger and is less easily damaged by acids and the wear and tear that can harm teeth.

On the other hand, when teeth are bathed in acidic saliva or corrosive foods and drinks, minerals flow out of the tooth, enamel crystals melt or dissolve, and the framework (the skeleton) becomes less densely packed, with smaller crystals. As the crystals melt (imagine an antacid tablet melting or dissolving in a glass of water) and become smaller, spaces or gaps, called *pores*, form between each crystal. As the spaces enlarge, they fill up with liquid. In this way, enamel under acidic attack loses its density and becomes more porous, and porous teeth are more likely to break, chip, or crumble. Porous teeth also stain more easily as colors from foods and drinks soak into their surface.

Understanding the difference fluoride can make to the outer shell of teeth explains why people with acidic mouths and damaged teeth should use dilute fluoride rinses to strengthen and protect them from any future acidity or dental damage.

When a dentist puts a white filling on the surface of a tooth he or she will etch the surface of that tooth with some acid, using this crystal "melting" process to purposefully remove minerals and open up pores in your tooth enamel so that he or she can attach the white filling material to the tooth surface. An acidic liquid is coated over the enamel and allowed to soak for a few seconds. The acidic liquid shrinks the enamel crystals and opens up pores between them. The acidic liquid is then washed away, and filling material is flowed onto the enamel and allowed to soak into the surface and into these microscopic holes. This method creates what appears to be (under the microscope) a mass of mini-fingers or tentacles clinging in the pore holes. To the patient, the white filling appears to magically stick onto the surface of the tooth. In fact, this has been a great demonstration of how quickly and easily tooth enamel crystals can be dissolved by acidity and how porous they make the tooth surface.

DEMINERALIZATION AND REMINERALIZATION

Dentists call the process of losing and gaining minerals in tooth enamel *demineralization* and *remineralization*. Demineralization occurs every time your mouth is acidic; the longer your mouth remains acidic, the more damage to your teeth. When enough minerals have dissolved, only the fragile skeleton of enamel will remain. Imagine a honeycomb without the honey. In this situation, any pressure or stress on the skeleton will cause it to break, forming a hole, or cavity. Despite the huge amount of fear, myth, and insecurity in many people's minds about cavities, there is only one way for a cavity to form. Acids in the mouth dissolve the strength of a tooth to the point at which it breaks.[7]

Remineralization is the rebuilding process that helps prevent a cavity.[8] The process occurs in almost everyone's mouth naturally but slowly, and the good news is that it can be speeded up by rinsing with fluoride or by regular exposure to xylitol. Remineralization repairs damaged enamel and can work to rebuild the tooth—sometimes completely, provided repairs begin before the enamel skeleton is physically broken. [9]

Our Teeth Are Sensitive

Weak or porous enamel can never adequately protect the live cells and nerves inside a tooth. Most people with acid-softened teeth notice their teeth are sensitive and hurt when they drink hot or cold beverages. The more porous your enamel, the more easily the inside of your tooth can be harmed. Damage to the nerve may be permanent and irreversible, resulting in the death of the tooth. When the nerve is damaged, treatment could require either root canal therapy and crowning or extraction and replacement of the tooth with implants or bridges. Keeping the outside of a tooth strong and remineralized is the key, not only to avoiding tooth pain and cavities, but also to extending the lifelong health of the inside of your teeth. Using products to strengthen and remineralize your teeth each day will provide protection to avoid cavities, fillings, repairs, and most of the dental treatments that people around you will experience as they age.

Throughout life, all the products we consume affect our teeth. Sometimes, acidic apple juice, sports drinks, sodas, coffee, and beer harm our teeth. At other times, our teeth may benefit from mineral-rich drinking water, vegetable juices, dairy products, xylitol, and alkaline soups and broths. The end state of your teeth—stained and weak or healthy and strong—is the final condition that results from the continuous swing between damage to your teeth and natural repair. Teeth will be sensitive and break when the damage outweighs the repairs. Teeth will be bright and strong if they are regularly able to rebuild themselves to full strength.

Many people who have cavities and bad teeth are those who, for whatever reason, do not have enough minerals in their saliva to provide the materials needed for this remineralization process. Some people have a dry mouth or insufficient saliva to coat, protect, and rebuild their teeth. Others find their own saliva tests acidic on a regular basis. Imagine having acidic saliva in your mouth all day and all night, weakening your teeth constantly and too acidic to offer protection from external acids from consumed foods or beverages. Such factors can quickly lead people into serious dental situations, with decay and cavities which could never be controlled by traditional flossing or dental cleanings. Dental problems in a dry mouth may actually be made worse with excessive toothbrushing or the frequent use of mouth rinses like Listerine, which itself has an acidity level capable of dissolving tooth enamel if it remains, undiluted, on teeth for a long period of time. (A beneficial way to use Listerine will be explained in detail as part of the complete dental care system described in part VI.)

The Dry Adolescent Mouth

Not long ago a young boy was sent to me by his dentist for evaluation. The boy had developed fifteen cavities, which his dentist said had suddenly appeared. Previous fillings were failing around the edges, his teeth were sensitive, and his gums were bleeding. This boy's dentist was worried about the number of new cavities and the fact that as soon as they were filled, more appeared. The boy's mother was concerned that the child was not eating well. The dentist and the mother were considering the possibility that the boy's soft teeth were symptoms of a calcium deficiency.

I sat the young man in my dental chair and examined his medical history and his damaged teeth. I talked to him about TV programs and, as we chatted, I asked which kind of soda he liked to drink. It turned out that he routinely took soda to bed and drank it while he watched his favorite late-night TV show. New braces made it impossible for the boy to close his mouth, which left his upper and lower front teeth completely unprotected and dry. Acidity from the soda promoted the growth of harmful bacteria which themselves produced more acidity as they multiplied, as well as poisons that caused gum irritation and bleeding. Compounding these problems were the hormonal changes of adolescence, which slow the flow and alter the chemistry of saliva, interfering with the natural healing of teeth. In his dry adolescent mouth, the soda and undiluted acids from harmful bacteria were destroying his teeth by direct contact and promoting a rampant dental disease that was attacking his gums and the tooth enamel all around his mouth. Poor toothbrushing made his situation worse and had allowed dangerous bacteria to multiply into thick, infected plaque that produced even more acidity and was damaging tooth enamel underneath the sticky layers.

The combination of all these factors created the most dentally dangerous conditions possible in the boy's mouth. With a dry mouth and adolescent hormonal changes, his natural repair process had virtually stopped. Without any balance from natural repair, only damage was occurring—damage from acidic drinks, harmful acid-producing bacteria, and acidic saliva. A calcium deficiency did not seem to be any real concern, and we decided to start addressing these obvious reasons by controlling the acidity that appeared responsible for the rapid tooth breakdown.

This situation shows how the perfect storm can trigger a progressive, destructive disease that escalates in severity without corrective help. It is also a clear example of how fillings cannot control dental disease.

The cavities on this teenager's teeth seemed to have appeared suddenly, but in fact the problems probably reached crisis point over some time before they were noticed. The acidic and dry conditions had allowed his teeth to be eroded and weakened all over his mouth until eventually fifteen teeth disintegrated at the same time. Enamel strength had dissolved over many months, possibly years. The tipping point had most likely been reached when braces were put on his teeth, drying his mouth even more and preventing any reversal of the damage by remineralization. The boy's potentially controllable problems were late-night snacking and poor oral hygiene, but his personality made me believe these habits would be difficult to change, so we needed to consider other options.

For this teenager the first home care priority was to have him use a mouth rinse that would help strengthen his teeth while he slept. A disinterested teen is more likely to rinse a couple of times a day with a good-tasting rinse than undertake complicated oral-care procedures such as flossing around braces. Selecting an appropriate rinse not only will serve to help strengthen tooth enamel but also will concentrate in plaque deposits and inactivate damaging bacteria. In addition to the rinse, I suggested some good-tasting xylitol mints which I knew he would like and a xylitol breath spray to help eradicate the harmful bacteria of dental disease. Within six months this boy's situation had noticeably improved; his teeth regained strength and his gums became healthier. Other rinses were added to his program and a shine began to show on the tooth enamel around his braces. Now was a good and appropriate time to fix any dental damage with fillings, and we could expect these new fillings to last longer than before.

Factors well beyond your control may have upset the delicate balance necessary to protect your teeth and may have left you vulnerable to cavities, plaque buildup, and continuous dental problems.[10] This situation needs to be controlled and the regular use of xylitol with special tooth-strengthening rinses will help people who may have tried other systems without success. With the extra help provided by these select products, patients with dry or acidic mouths often gain control over their dental problems and bring an end to their ongoing and expensive dental treatments.

While we sleep, all of us have less saliva and drier, more acidic mouth conditions than during the day. Consequently, our teeth are at increased risk during the night. The extra dryness in our mouths makes it vitally important that we use a balanced and protective oral-care routine every night before going to sleep and ideally again in the morning at the start of our day.

CHAPTER FIVE

Mouth Chemistry

In a healthy mouth, your teeth are bathed in a thin, watery liquid called *saliva*. When saliva becomes acidic, even temporarily, it has the potential to dissolve minerals from the outer enamel that covers your teeth. When tooth minerals dissolve away, your teeth will become weaker and more porous, more sensitive to temperature, and more easily stained.

The chemistry of your saliva can change for many reasons (see the list in chapter 3). Sometimes those changes in salivary acidity are temporary; sometimes they are more permanent. Changes can sometimes be intense, as when gastric acid enters the mouth with acid reflux or from soft drinks; citric, apple, and grape juices; or frozen fruit juice in beverages or ice pops. Research has shown that frozen juices cause the greatest mouth acidity, and refrigerated fruit juices are more damaging than those drunk at room temperature.[1]

Acid-producing mouth bacteria also increase overall mouth acidity, but the place where these bacteria lodge, close against the tooth surface, is usually where there is the greatest acid concentration and therefore the greatest chance of tooth damage. Such areas are between teeth (where teeth touch each other) and inside the pits and grooves on biting surfaces of molar teeth.

Acidic or Alkaline Saliva

In a healthy, normal mouth, chewing and eating foods stimulates nonacidic saliva flow. Saliva is produced by glands in cheek tissues, under the jaw, and all around the skin inside your mouth. Saliva helps us digest food and also washes away food particles stuck on teeth and gums. One of the greatest dental benefits of healthy saliva is that it contains minerals necessary for rebuilding the strength of enamel. Nonacidic—that is, neutral, or *alkaline*—saliva also dilutes acidic liquids in your mouth and around your teeth. In these ways, saliva makes its contribution as an acid-reducing system and a tooth-protecting mechanism essential for tooth health. The greater amount of healthy saliva you have in your mouth, the more tooth cleansing, remineralization, and protection you will have.

The consistency or thickness of saliva is also important for tooth health because saliva is needed to lubricate teeth. Whenever you clench your teeth or chew, the lubrication of saliva on opposite surfaces prevents damaging them. In a dry mouth, teeth can become severely worn, just as parts of a car engine might be if they ran without oil.

Saliva flow varies for every person and also at different times of the day. It increases at mealtimes and slows down while we sleep. Without saliva, there is little protection for teeth and, in a dry mouth, little or no natural repair. Consequently, tooth enamel can become especially vulnerable and quickly damaged.

If you have upper or lower front teeth that are not covered by your lips because your lips are thin or perhaps your teeth are longer, those teeth will be drier and less protected than other teeth. Any teeth that are dry and not bathed in the saliva of your mouth will be at greater risk for cavities and dental problems. Many toddlers and small children have lips that do not close completely, and their teeth are often dry and unprotected, especially while they sleep. Dentists call this problem *incomplete lip closure*, and patients with front teeth that are often or always exposed to the air become very dry because they are not bathed in saliva in the normal way. Cavities form quickly on the smooth front and back surfaces of these dry and unprotected teeth, unless special care is taken to protect them.

Thus, the *amount* of saliva is just as important as the *acidity level* of saliva for the health of your teeth. Laboratory tests such as the Saliva-Check Buffer Kit made by GC America can tell whether you have less saliva than normal and can analyze its chemistry. The rate at which saliva flows into the mouth can also be measured using CRT bacteria and Dentocult laboratory testing. Such tests may be used for people who have a severely dry mouth because of disease or radiation damage, but most people are aware if their mouth feels dry.

Even in a dry mouth, however, there are a variety of ways to increase salivary flow and help ensure that adequate minerals are available for building and strengthening teeth. Building tooth strength benefits your teeth the same way strength training increases bone density in order to resist osteoporosis, fractures, and other bone problems in later life.

Acidity and Tooth Damage

When I give talks, I usually take a couple of eggs with me to demonstrate the corrosiveness of acid, because an eggshell in many ways resembles the enamel shell of teeth. The night before the talk, I immerse these uncooked eggs in an acidic liquid, which, I explain, is like soaking your teeth in something acidic. Vinegar works well for the eggshell experiment, but you could use any acidic liquid to dissolve the eggshells. My audience is usually shocked when I show them how the acidity has removed the hard outer coating of the egg and made the shell soft and easily rubbed away. Next I drop the egg into a cup of coffee or a tumbler of grape juice or wine. The porous acid-softened shell quickly becomes dark and stained. I explain how acids have a similar effect on teeth and how acid-softened enamel stains quickly and easily.

To tell whether or not a liquid is acidic you can measure its pH. A pH measurement can be taken with litmus paper or, if a more accurate measurement is needed, with a special pH meter. A pH meter has a small tube-shaped probe that looks like a thermometer attached to a computerized gauge. The gauge is calibrated to give very accurate pH measurements as the probe is dipped into test liquids. The score, or pH reading, instantly shows on the screen as a digital number. A pH meter is probably more sensitive than you need for testing the acidity of everyday foods and drinks, and it's a relatively expensive piece of equipment, but it is fun to use at lectures.

Litmus paper, on the other hand, is inexpensive and can be purchased on the Internet or at health food stores.[2] Different papers have different ranges of sensitivity; you need a range between pH 5 and 8 for the mouth. A pH testing kit includes paper and a color chart so you can interpret your results. When litmus paper is moistened or dipped into a liquid, the paper changes to a color that reflects the chemistry of the liquid. You match the paper against a chart to find a similar color and find its corresponding pH number, which is the acidity measurement for the test liquid.

A pH scale is an imaginary scale numbered between 1 and 14. An alkaline liquid, such as milk, would have a high number, somewhere between 7 and 14. The more alkaline the liquid, the higher the number and the pH. An acidic liquid, such as vinegar, would have a low number, always lower than the neutral pH 7. The more acidic the liquid, the lower the number and the pH. A reading that comes out just below pH 5.5, for example, would indicate that the liquid could severely damage tooth enamel because minerals dissolve out of tooth enamel crystals in a mouth with that pH level, thereby weakening teeth in much the same way that the eggshells were dissolved.

Once my audience understands that low pH numbers are acidic and that acidity can cause damage to teeth, I walk around and collect samples from the various drinks people have selected to sip during the event. I line up the samples on my demonstration table and dip my pH measuring gauge into each one. The selection includes a variety of beverages and bottled waters routinely consumed in the United States. I measure soda, sports drinks, iced teas, diet drinks, and more. Apple juice usually horrifies the audience with its pH of around 2.2. Suddenly people see the importance of knowing the acidity of the liquids they are putting into their mouths.

TEST YOUR SALIVA

Saliva pH measurements can be used to visually monitor how quickly changes occur in the mouth and how saliva acidity can change in different life situations. Ideally, you should take a mouth acidity (pH) reading in the morning, right after you wake up. This will give you a recording that is independent of changes caused by eating or drinking.

Begin the test by spitting a small amount of saliva into a spoon and dipping a strip of litmus paper (or a litmus stick) into the liquid. If you test your resting or morning saliva and find it is neutral or alkaline, you will generally have good salivary protection for your teeth. If you find your saliva is acidic, you may be at higher risk for cavities and tooth decay.[3] A truly healthy mouth ideally has a resting acidity measurement of close to pH 7. Any time your mouth's acidity level falls below the number 6, you should be worried about your teeth.

Test your saliva again during the day after drinking something acidic (coffee; grape, apple, or cranberry juice; or lemonade). Compare the new pH reading to the baseline early-morning litmus test of your resting saliva pH to see how the drink changed your saliva to become more acidic. Now test again at ten-minute intervals and see how long it takes for your mouth to return to your baseline state.

In a healthy mouth with plenty of natural saliva, a neutral pH usually returns within half an hour. The length of time varies for different people, but your test will give you a picture of how efficiently your saliva copes with an acidic attack. People with quicker recovery times, whose saliva rapidly returns their mouth to normal, will obviously have more protection for their teeth and less time for any tooth damage.[4]

Enamel crystals dissolve out of teeth faster and faster as mouth acidity increases. Worse, the damage increases by a factor of ten with each single-unit drop in acidity. This means that having a really acidic mouth will seriously damage your teeth. Some of the most acidic liquids in the mouth are stomach acids, which is especially important to know if you have acid reflux disease or bulimia. It is also important to be aware that many carbonated sodas and sports drinks (diet just as much as regular) are very acidic (as low as pH 2.2) and therefore damaging to teeth, regardless of their sugar content. People who drink a lot of soda or acidic sports and juice beverages should realize that their teeth are being soaked during each gulp in something extremely damaging and corrosive.

Holistic medical practitioners believe it is important to control general body acidity for overall health. Basically, the belief is that germs are less able to grow in and take over an alkaline body, and the more acidic your body, the more disease prone you become. In death, our bodies are completely acidic, which allows our bodies to be over-taken by bacteria and decompose.

Louis Pasteur, famous for his role in preventing disease with vaccination and pasteurization, is said to have uttered on his deathbed, "It is not the germ; it is the terrain." What Pasteur and others were saying, as early as the 1900s, was that they recognized the importance of the body's vulnerability and also the factors that could build resistance to disease. The same is true for the mouth. If you reduce the acidity in your mouth and try to control the growth of acid-loving bacteria, your mouth will be a more hostile place for harmful disease bacteria and instead will be a place where your teeth will remain healthy and strong.

CREATE AN ALKALINE BALANCE

Holistic doctors encourage us to eat herbs, fresh vegetables, fruits, vitamins, and minerals to create an alkaline balance in the body. Alkalizing your body is a little more complicated than alkalizing your mouth, but the foods that work for your body will generally work for your mouth. Potatoes, asparagus, and broccoli, for example, leave saliva alkaline. The biggest difference from holistic medicine is that vinegar and lemon juice—often used to control acid reflux and promoted for alkalizing the body—are acidic liquids that can damage tooth enamel if not washed away. Steps should always be taken to quickly remove the acidity of citrus juices and vinegar from around teeth.

Most men suffer dental damage as their saliva dries up because of age, mouth-drying medications, or breathing with their mouth open, especially at night.[5] Women, on the other hand, often find they have acidic saliva during pregnancy, during hormonal changes, and even as they enter their mid-to-late thirties. Thus, women have to worry more about fighting mouth acidity than men do.

Like many women who multitask in their busy lives, I am prone to an acidic mouth and am aware of the damage this could cause to my teeth and possibly my health. Measuring the pH of my saliva has shown me how it becomes more alkaline about half an hour after I have taken vitamins, when I relax in a sauna, or when I bask on the beach during vacation. Many forms of relaxation, including gardening and exercising, likewise seem to have positive alkalizing effects on my saliva. (And I find it easy to assume that the things that alkalize my mouth may benefit my general health as well.)

People need to realize that there is no single salivary pH and that one reading that shows a normal pH is not a guarantee that it will remain healthy. Regular readings will help you determine how much protection you have naturally for your teeth and when you may want to be particularly careful during times of more mouth acidity.

Avoid Acidity

Anyone's saliva can quickly turn acidic without warning and create an acidic mouth environment that can cause long-lived or temporary damage to teeth. As we've seen previously, the trigger for this change can be anything from a stressful business meeting to family problems to a situation as serious as bereavement. Even the anticipation of a dental appointment may cause a change in the pH of your saliva. Anyone who is familiar with public speaking or theater knows how saliva thickens right before the show begins. Saliva alters in quality and quantity because of a natural reaction to stress and returns to normal after the event. Most people will have noticed how speakers keep water nearby, because their mouths naturally become dry and their saliva thicker.

Many changes in salivary acidity are temporary, lasting only until the situation or stress has gone, but sometimes saliva remains acidic for longer periods, even months or years. People who are depressed, under stress, or dealing with emotional problems should be aware that their teeth may be at increased risk for acidic damage. The last thing any of these people need at times like these is a cascade of dental problems to add to their trials and tribulations.

People with acidic mouths, or anyone who believes his or her mouth may be acidic, should work even harder to protect their teeth from this acidic damage. Acidity can also be caused by illness, poor nutrition, chemotherapy, lack of sunshine, depression, medications, or hormonal imbalances that may include pregnancy. In relaxed environments, with regained physical and emotional health, saliva pH will usually return to normal again.

Some people find themselves with acidic saliva no matter what they do. This can happen as people age, for those with acid reflux, or those who are chronically sick or dying. Patients with acid reflux have strong stomach acids that enter the mouth at frequent intervals, and this attack almost always occurs when patients lie down to sleep. Acids in the mouth at this time can remain on teeth for hours if they are not washed away by saliva. Consequently, the worst tooth damage from acid reflux will take place in a dry mouth. This may be the mouth of someone who snores, takes mouth-drying medications, or simply sleeps with the mouth wide open.[6]

Harmful acid-producing mouth germs can themselves generate mouth acidity, especially when those germs multiply and grow in a dry mouth or when they have frequent access to sugary or high carbohydrate food or drink ingredients. Harmful germs not only thrive in an acidic mouth but also constantly produce acids that increase the generalized acidity of the mouth. When teeth are coated with unhealthy germs, acidity levels may be sufficient to weaken and damage tooth surfaces all over the mouth, but particularly under the plaque layer itself.

For most healthy people, the main source of damaging mouth acidity is from frequent and intermittent consumption of acidic foods and beverages. Whatever the cause, an acidic mouth increases your risk for dental problems, brittle teeth, sensitivity, broken fillings, tooth wear, and gum disease, and the damage will always be worse when combined with mouth dryness or lack of saliva.

Ideally, you should not eat or drink before going to bed, because food residue can remain on your teeth for hours. Some people imagine that diet drinks or sugarless cookies will be safe for teeth before bed. Diet drinks are extremely acidic and will often cause severe damage if consumed before sleeping. Any detrimental liquid can remain in tooth crevices and grooves during the night, causing erosion, weakening, and damage. On the other hand, if you leave something beneficial on your teeth before going to bed, it can linger in these crevices or between teeth and may help to repair and remineralize teeth, actually making them stronger while you sleep!

Children's Saliva

Children usually have saliva that quickly restores their mouths to an alkaline state after sugary candy or an acidic drink. This gives protection to their teeth, provided there is sufficient recovery time between acid attacks. For that reason, it is important to limit nibbling on sugary candy or sipping acidic drinks. Even in small quantities, these snacks will be more damaging to teeth than consuming larger servings less often. Sucking sugary lollipops and ring pops or sipping on juice-filled boxes or cups can create major dental problems for children. If the idea of stopping these habits is difficult to imagine, use tooth-protective foods and xylitol to interrupt the acidity of the nibbling or sipping cycle and help protect teeth from the damage such sugary and acidic things can cause.

Years ago when my children returned from Halloween trick-or-treating, we sat together on the floor and ate candy—as much as was reasonable at one time. At the end of the session, we finished with a tooth-protective food, such as an apple, a stalk of celery, or something dairy. It was always a fun-filled time for us and a better alternative than picking slowly at a bag of forbidden sweets. Today I encourage parents to remember that gum or candy made with 100 percent xylitol is another perfect Halloween treat, especially at the end of a sweet-treat evening. And, although it is possible to bake with xylitol, I personally prefer traditional desserts and use xylitol as a refreshing breath mint to complete a meal.

Saliva and Aging

As we age, saliva's ability to protect teeth becomes weaker or non-existent, especially for elderly women and those on medications. A frequent side effect of medications is a dry mouth and reduced saliva flow. Sweetened liquid diets may remain on teeth, not only damaging enamel but also making the mouth acidic. More than ever, people in their midlife should work to strengthen their teeth and protect them day and night. One of the first places to notice damage is on the outside surface of back molar teeth. Pieces of enamel chip away where teeth bend and flex, creating a groove close to the gum line. Many patients mistakenly think that careless brushing causes this groove, but it is often the first sign of an acidic mouth and should be a signal that, without help, more damage may be on its way. The groove can expose the root surfaces of back teeth, making them sensitive to temperature changes and touch. If acidic damage continues, the edges of fillings will flake away next, causing the fillings to loosen, leak, and finally fail.

I often catch the attention of my seminar audience by describing this predictable chain of events that most often occurs in the mouths of women during midlife. It will happen in any mouth attacked by acidity. Because the damage occurs in a sequence, I can describe how the patients first notice sensitive back teeth and fillings that start to fail and need replacement, followed by root-canal treatments and crowns to repair the damage. Once all this work is finished, gums become the next target, requiring extra cleaning visits, scaling, and deep cleaning. Finally there will be extractions for the teeth that can no longer be saved, and maybe implants, bridges, or dentures to replace them. The sad part is that with some proactive steps, this damage could have been prevented and tooth damage averted.

You may be able to trace your own dental problems to dry mouth, mouth acidity, acidic beverages and snacks, or acid reflux. The drier your mouth, the longer acidity will be able to remain on your teeth. People with nasal blockage from allergies or asthma find their dry mouths often cause dental problems. Weak teeth, damaged by mouth acids, will not be able to resist the pressure of biting and chewing, and without help, pieces of enamel will chip off under the slightest stress.

It is staggering to realize that almost all American adults have damage from dental disease as they age, and almost a quarter of all adults between sixty-five and seventy-four have severe disease. In the United States today, around 30 percent of adults age sixty-five have no teeth at all. Many people, despite visits to their dentist, are never cured of their disease, but they continue to require treatments year after year, with repairs becoming constantly more extensive. Dental visits are often a maintenance system that does not stop the disease but, rather, simply keeps the symptoms within limits that you, the consumer, agree to accept. Patients have been conditioned to view fillings and repairs as normal, as problems that are part of the aging process, and their ongoing dental treatments as something they deserve. On the contrary, I expect that with the repeated and consistent use of my system, my teeth will not deteriorate over time, but will remain healthy and even become healthier, brighter, and stronger over the years ahead.

Dental damage can sometimes creep up on people as a nasty surprise. Those who have never experienced a filling or gum problem may find that a life change of some kind precipitates a domino effect of dental disasters. One sensitive tooth, a cavity that needs filling, weakened enamel, a repair that leads to a root-canal treatment, and finally a crown. The story is painful to hear, because so often this damage could have easily been prevented.[7]

PART THREE

Gum Health

Dentists have the obligation of making the results and benefits of their investigative efforts available to all when they are useful in safeguarding or promoting the health of the public.

—ADA Principles and Ethics Code of Professional Conduct

CHAPTER SIX

Plaque

In 1890 German engineer W. D. Miller worked with Dr. G. V. Black to learn more about cavities in teeth. Using a microscope, Miller noticed a connection between bacteria in the mouth and a film that appeared to cover teeth; he named the layer *dental plaque*. Miller and Black remain famous today for helping dentistry become both a science and a profession. Their accounts are interesting to read and stand up well in the light of today's knowledge.[1]

Dental plaque became linked with tooth decay in the 1900s. This was an exciting time for scientists because so many new medical discoveries were being made. Antibiotics had been discovered, and people were learning that medicines could kill germs and prevent disease. Medicines enabled doctors to stop or control sickness in a way that had not been possible before. In the climate of that time, all germs were considered bad and viewed as carriers of infection and disease. In the early days of antibiotics, treatments were designed to kill as many germs as possible, regardless of their kind. Many years later, doctors and scientists realized that when all bacteria are destroyed, unexpected and sometimes very undesirable side effects can occur.

Germs Protect

Today we have become comfortable with the concept that many germs live inside and outside healthy bodies and do us no harm—in fact, many of them provide health benefits. Healthy germs protect our bodies, and if they disappear or are removed, we may experience digestive problems, poor absorption of vitamins, and even overgrowth of bad germs or fungus. Few people have considered that it is similar in a healthy mouth, where protective bacteria work to control yeast infections and overgrowth of the harmful bacteria of dental disease. It is understandable that, in the atmosphere of the 1900s, doctors of early dentistry believed all mouth germs were bad and thought that the film on teeth, where the bacteria were found, should be eliminated for teeth to be healthy.

In the Middle Ages, people believed that holes in teeth were caused by a worm that ate through them. Although no one today believes that cavities are caused by worms, many incorrect ideas about cavities and plaque remain in people's minds. Most people still cling to the idea that plaque is bad, and have never considered that a healthy film over teeth has benefits to protect enamel and keep teeth strong and comfortable.

In fact, an intricate interplay exists among the many kinds of bacteria that live in the misunderstood and often feared *biofilm* that forms naturally over the surface of our teeth. This film or healthy plaque is not leftover food stuck between your teeth, but a delicate mesh of proteins and other materials harboring a neighborhood of living bacteria. Plaque is a complicated mixture of many kinds of bacteria, protein strands, other substances, fluids, and cells. In its healthiest state it is a unique microcosm, a community of cells that thrive together in an organized way. Plaque is described as having a group character, which gives it extraordinary resistance to temperatures and corrosive liquids that foods and drinks bring to our mouths and that would otherwise kill individual cells at much lower concentrations. It may surprise the reader to learn that the components of healthy plaque have unique properties that allow it to protect the underlying tooth. Removing this natural protection can leave tooth enamel unprotected and at possible risk for chemical and thermal damage and potentially harmful infection.

When I ask patients how they imagine cavities form, the main word in their reply is almost always "plaque," yet few can explain why. People believe that the priority for preventing cavities is to clean plaque off teeth as often and as thoroughly as possible. Almost no one has considered the possibility that teeth may not need regular cleanings if plaque is maintained in a state of total health.

Healthy Plaque

Patients view plaque as an enemy beyond their control, gluing to teeth like barnacles stick to the hull of a ship. They believe that the scraping chisels of a dental hygienist are needed to fight this mythological demon. Many believe hygienists exist mainly for the purpose of eliminating plaque. The truth is that healthy plaque may be essential for maintaining clean, strong teeth. Healthy plaque fights away intruding bacteria, provides essential ingredients for enamel to heal itself, and also protects vital cells from temperature and chemical changes that occur during eating and drinking.

In order for teeth to remain healthy, comfortable, and cavity free you need to develop and maintain protective plaque on your teeth. Instead of striving to remove every vestige of plaque from teeth with aggressive chemicals and abrasives, it may be more valuable to assess, test, monitor, and adjust the surface film on your teeth to ensure that it is healthy.

In 2005 I was fortunate enough to be at a dental conference where pictures of plaque were magnified on video monitors for all of us to see in detail from our chairs.[2] Examining the composition of plaque made me realize how its removal without cause may be more harmful than we have imagined. The monitors showed that the cells in plaque communicate and depend on each other, with waste products from one providing food for another. We could see cells moving about in groups, encased in bubble-shaped spaces. Other cells were on their own, working their way between the fibers like spiders in a web. Liquids and foods could pass through the plaque layers to reach bacteria deep inside. In thin layers of healthy plaque, air was also able to flow in and out among the layers.[3]

I think of healthy plaque as a kind of bed comforter that will cover and protect your teeth. Imagine that bed bugs invade the inside of your comforter. Suddenly you have a very different situation, and the comforter is no longer protective but a source of risk and damage. Imagine if the bugs produced harmful liquids that could seep through the quilt and harm you.

I would suggest that instead of depending on dental professionals removing the film of plaque from your teeth sporadically, it would be better to focus on maintaining the health of good tooth plaque every day. Harmful germs must be prevented from infecting this film, and from multiplying. As harmful plaque bacteria mature, they change in nature, and some can form noxious liquids that damage teeth and gums. Harmful bacteria appear to grow in tightly packed rows which form overlapping layers, creating a barrier that prevents oxygen from reaching the deeper layers. Especially harmful to teeth are so-called *anaerobic plaque bacteria*, which grow in low-oxygen areas. Anaerobic bacteria are usually found close to the tooth surface, deeply buried under layers of infected plaque. These bacteria are very aggressive and produce quantities of acid that causes extreme harm to teeth as it seeps out and attacks the tooth surface underneath.

In the early 1970s dentists noticed that if infected plaque was not brushed away from teeth, the white, foamy layer grew thicker each day. As plaque layers thicken, the tooth surface under them slowly changes color. When tooth enamel has been covered with infected plaque for three weeks, the tooth surface underneath it turns white. When this plaque layer is wiped away, the shape of the white area on the tooth surface corresponds exactly to the shape of the area previously covered by the plaque.[4] Called *white spot infections*, these areas develop consistently every twenty-one days when infected plaque, fueled with starch or sugar from the diet, is not cleaned off a tooth surface. After twenty-one days, the weakened tooth begins to crumble and cave in, and a cavity will result.

Working from this observation, the Karlstad program of 1974 was born.[5] The program was based on the idea that if plaque could be removed before the twenty-first day, cavities would never form. The hypothesis was that cavities could not form if three things occurred: (1) patients controlled their sugar intake; (2) they received fluoride treatments; and (3) plaque was removed regularly (definitely before the twenty-first day). Because the researchers had little confidence in patients' ability to clean their teeth, specially trained staff gave the participants tooth cleanings at three-week intervals. The interval between cleanings was later extended to three months, and in this way the idea of hygienists giving periodic professional cleanings was born and has been followed ever since. Interestingly, the Karlstad study showed that despite sugar control, fluoride, and cleanings, cavities were not completely prevented.

Dental Cleaning

Until the 1980s, the term *dental cleaning* applied to cleaning away any hardened deposits from teeth and polishing the teeth with brushes and pastes. Today, a cleaning refers to a simple polishing of the teeth, and the removal of hard deposits is referred to as *periodontal treatment*.

There is no doubt that if you have a buildup of hardened plaque around the edges of your teeth, its removal with periodontal treatments will reduce gum irritation and offer you a better chance of regaining gum health. Dental tools are designed to scrape and dislodge this hardened, infected crust from between teeth and from above and under the gums. Most people know the areas in their mouth where this calcified deposit is likely to form. The calcified layer can irritate the gums and attract bacteria and food that easily stick to it. When your mouth becomes healthy and your mouth acidity is balanced, plaque will not be infected and you will begin to notice that these calcified deposits will be reduced in amount and may ultimately stop forming.

Today in almost every dental office across the USA, a patient has a dental cleaning at each recall visit, at least twice each year. These treatments are prescribed without any evaluation to determine if this cleaning is necessary. Very few dentists question whether their patients would have better dental health without a cleaning. Obviously, too much polishing will damage the dense and most protective outer layer of a tooth and disrupt any delicate protective plaque layer on the tooth surface. Any polishing that removes this dense layer of enamel from your tooth makes teeth more porous. In this way a cleaning may potentially cause teeth to become more sensitive and more easily stained and can possibly open the surface to infection.

In the early 1970s a study was carried out on U.S. Navy recruits that showed the protective nature of plaque. The study illustrated how healthy plaque acts as a defense against unwanted bacteria and how cleaning it away could expose healthy teeth to infection.[6] The recruits were separated into two groups: those with cavities and cavity-forming bacteria in their mouths and those with healthy teeth free of harmful bacteria.

Half the recruits in each of the two groups were given a professional dental cleaning. Every recruit was asked to rinse with a liquid that contained cavity-forming bacteria. The recruits were then tested for the presence of harmful bacteria in their mouths. Researchers were surprised to find that the recruits with healthy teeth—but who had received a cleaning—were now infected with cavity-forming bacteria. The only remaining group with healthy mouths was the group of recruits who came with healthy teeth and did not receive a cleaning.

Twenty years after this forgotten experiment, a researcher named P. D. Marsh proposed in 1994 that in order for a mouth to be truly healthy, the bacteria in it need to be healthy. Marsh's theory states that removal of plaque in a healthy mouth is not necessary.[7] He looked closely at the kinds of bacteria living in plaque and believed that harmful ones multiply and cause disease only under certain conditions. Marsh was confident that harmful germs exist only when a shift in mouth chemistry encourages acid-producing bacteria to grow. Marsh believed that in a healthy mouth, bacteria do not need to be removed because they are, in fact, healthy and protective.[8]

The public has been conditioned to believe that dental cleanings are for the benefit of their teeth. The truth is that professional cleanings may reduce deposits, but they cannot stop the regrowth of acid-loving bacteria, and cleanings themselves cannot strengthen or protect your teeth. As you exit the dental office after a cleaning, any harmful bacteria present in your saliva will already be reestablishing themselves on your teeth. No amount of brushing, flossing, or professional cleanings can completely rid your mouth of bacteria. These treatments may remove a number of the bacteria, but no matter how well your teeth are cleaned, they will never be clean from a microbiological point of view. Some bacteria will always be left behind. Unless you remove the conditions that promote harmful bacterial problems, more harmful bacteria will grow back and any cycle of damage will be repeated.

The fewer acid-forming germs there are in plaque, the less acid will be produced and, correspondingly, the less damage to teeth. Healthy, alkaline plaque will not cause demineralization and damage, and healthy bacteria are not sticky, so they are more easily removed from teeth with simple brushing and rinsing. The best plan is to create an environment where healthy bacteria thrive. How can someone achieve this? The simplest way is to avoid mouth acidity as much as possible and to encourage healthy plaque by consuming sufficient 100 percent xylitol each day, especially after meals and beverages. Over time, you will have less buildup of plaque, and you will notice your teeth and gums become healthier—with or without dental cleanings.

At least 6-10 grams of xylitol per day is recommended in (at least 5-6) divided doses. Mints, gum, breath sprays or granular xylitol are all acceptable. My general recommendation is to dissolve one teaspoon of granulated xylitol in 6-8 ounces of water and drink this each morning. This can be repeated again in the afternoon, or mints and gum can be eaten at the end of snacks or meals. Using this xylitol regimen is an easy way to ensure sufficient dosage (one teaspoon = 4 grams) and multiple, separate exposures. Frequency is believed to play a major role in reducing plaque.

Also, remember to clean and disinfect toothbrushes and household eating utensils to eliminate the transfer of harmful bacteria between family members.

CHAPTER SEVEN

Gum Disease

Dentists talk about two kinds of gum disease—gingivitis and periodontitis—although the latter (which I discuss in detail later in this
chapter) is really just a more serious version that develops from the
former.

Gingivitis

Mild inflammation of the gums is called *gingivitis,* and it affects as
many as one in seven adults, even those who routinely visit their dentist.[1] Almost all senior citizens with natural teeth have mild, moderate, or severe gingivitis that becomes worse as they age. Sometimes
the only sign is gum recession or exposure of the roots of teeth, which

many people accept as natural or unavoidable with age. Why do so many people have gum diseases? Most dentists would answer that people do not floss enough, although perhaps it is because most people have the conditions that promote unhealthy plaque as they age. Aging adults generally have moderate to severe mouth acidity and frequently a dry mouth to complicate the condition.

Each tooth stands inside a hole in the jaw known as the tooth socket. Between the surface of the tooth and this tooth socket there is a small gap. A healthy tooth is attached to the jawbone by little fibers that look like small hairs running from the tooth surface across a space and into the jawbone. You can see that the surface of the tooth below the gum line is different from the part of the tooth visible in the mouth. The root surface is covered with softer cement that transforms to hard enamel as the tooth becomes visible in the mouth. The place where cement and enamel meet is called the *cementoenamel junction.*

In a healthy mouth, the gums hug the tooth tightly at this junction, like an elastic collar gripping the neck of the tooth. This tight gum collar keeps bacteria and food particles from entering the gap under its surface. The gum collar also protects the soft cement–coated root of the tooth from contact with liquids and temperature changes that occur during eating and drinking. If this gum collar becomes infected, it can swell, bleed, and possibly loosen its grip on the teeth. Liquids and air can then seep down the space to irritate the soft, unprotected root surface beneath the gum line. Acidic liquids easily damage vulnerable root cement, and if cold air touches this surface, the person feels excruciating pain. Although the real problem is the health of your gums, the symptoms show up as sensitivity of the teeth to hot and cold.

Few people realize how easy it is to treat gingivitis with the home remedies of good tooth cleaning and the correct use of mouth rinses as prescribed in my regimen. Harmful germs in plaque cause gum infections, and harmful bacteria flourish in acidic and dry mouths.

Removing bacteria by good brushing, cleaning your toothbrush every time you brush, using my suggested rinse system, and consuming adequate amounts of xylitol can completely cure gingivitis in a matter of days.

Mild gum disease is usually not painful, and if you successfully clean the infected area, the bleeding stops quickly. When the gum area is clean, the swelling will go down without causing any permanent damage to your gums or your teeth. It is important to brush bleeding gums as soon as you notice any problem. If cold water makes your teeth hurt, use warm water on your toothbrush. If using a brush is too painful at first, wipe some gauze or a clean piece of cloth over your gums. Use the mouth rinses in the special sequence I recommend, and remember to clean your toothbrush, since bacteria can grow and flourish on it.

Unfortunately, most people are worried about making their gums bleed, so they avoid a bleeding area, allowing the gingivitis to progress and become worse, slowly developing into the next and more advanced stage. At this more advanced stage the bleeding may stop, but this is not a good sign, because it may indicate that the first stage of gingivitis is now progressing deeper down the sides of the tooth beneath the gums.

Some people suggest remedies for gingivitis that involve brushing with baking soda or rinsing with hydrogen peroxide. These remedies may be useful for a limited period of time, but frequent use of baking soda and peroxide seems to sensitize gum tissue for many people and result in gum recession. Anyone devoted to the use of baking soda or peroxide should consider taking probiotics. My concern is that these products eliminate not only harmful plaque, but also the healthy, protective biofilm we need for oral health. I recommend that people use a sequence of mouth rinses that work a particular magic because of their effect on the biology and chemistry of the teeth when they are used together in a specific order. (My complete dental care system is described in part VI.)

When harmful plaque bacteria have been cleaned away from your teeth and gums, it will take only a few days for gingivitis to heal itself and the damage to be reversed. Look constantly for bleeding or puffy gums in your mouth, and if you notice them, check that you have cleaned your toothbrush, begin extra brushing, and make sure you eat adequate amounts of xylitol to immediately help reverse the damage.

Periodontitis

More advanced gum disease is called *periodontitis,* and it can be graded as mild, moderate, or severe. If the gum area around the neck of your teeth is allowed to remain infected for too long, it can lose its elasticity. The collar that normally grips tightly around the tooth breaks away, opening up a space called a pocket. This pocket provides a protected home for bacteria and other mouth debris, which gradually move deeper into the pocket and force their way down the root of your tooth. The bacteria that live in a periodontal pocket are more aggressive than the kind normally found on teeth. Some of them create reactions in the adjacent gum tissues which can destroy the fibers that hold teeth inside the jaws. As these fibers are destroyed, the pocket increases in size and depth, making it ever more difficult to clean with just rinsing and toothbrushes.

Periodontitis becomes difficult to reverse once the pocket is too deep to reach with a toothbrush bristle to clean inside it. When a dentist measures the depth of a pocket around your teeth, he or she will be concerned as soon as a depth of four millimeters is reached. This is because four millimeters is the length of a toothbrush bristle. Although I do not recommend this, sometimes people try cleaning machines such as the Waterpik, which blasts a power spray into this pocket in an attempt to clean the deeper areas. Although most periodontal specialists will be skeptical, I suggest anyone with deep pockets try vigorous 2–3 minute rinsing with unflavored Closys, the first cleansing rinse in my complete mouth care system. I have heard of 10-millimeter pockets dramatically improving when all the parts of my system have been used conscientiously over a period of several months.

Damage can progress quickly once the bacteria of periodontitis start to multiply in pockets, gradually destroying more and more tooth-connecting fibers. Although people usually feel no pain at this stage, they may start to notice a bad taste in their mouth or have constant bad breath because food particles and infection also build up in the pocket. Some patients nevertheless do feel a dull, throbbing pain which is from inflammation and buildup of infection in the confined area of the tooth socket. Pressure from liquids and bacteria press on the jawbone and may gradually cause it to erode away, leaving the tooth without bony support. Abscesses and infection can make a tooth too sensitive for chewing. This kind of severe infection may progress to the end of the root. At this stage the disease is terminal for a tooth. Sadly, in most cases this pain and suffering could have been avoided or arrested and reversed if adequately treated during the first stages of gingivitis, when the gums were just slightly infected and simply bleeding.

Dental Health and General Health

A hundred years ago, dentists believed that it was important to rid the body of infection by extracting suspicious teeth. They believed in a theory called *the focus of infection*, which implicated bad teeth as a cause of severe and general medical problems. Once again, medical doctors have become suspicious of infection in the mouth and often ask dentists to check the jaws of their patients to find any dead teeth or areas of infection when unexplained diseases occur or before difficult major surgery is to be performed.

Indeed, in the past ten years many direct and often surprising connections have been made between dental health and general health. Gum disease has been linked not only to heart problems (see the discussion "Gum Disease and Bacterial Endocarditis" that follows) but also to high blood pressure, risk of stroke, insulin instability for diabetic patients, infertility treatment failure, and the risk of preterm birth.[2] (See details in the section "Gum Disease and Preterm Births" later in this chapter.) The latest information is best accessed online at the ADA's website and related medical ones.

Scientists at the Harvard School of Public Health in Boston have shown recently that gum disease may be linked to pancreatic cancer.[3] Pancreatic cancer affects more than 33,000 Americans each year and kills more than 30,000, making it the fourth leading cause of death from cancer. Researchers say the findings need to be confirmed by additional research, but after taking into consideration such factors as age, smoking, diabetes, and body mass index, men with gum disease were 63 percent more likely to develop pancreatic cancer than those without gum disease. In the nonsmoking group, men with gum disease were twice as likely as those with healthy gums to develop this hard-to-treat cancer.

Although we do not yet have definitive proof, there are indications that oral bacteria may be involved in other body infections, including irritable bowel syndrome and related intestinal problems. Others believe that there may be a dental connection with conditions such as rheumatoid arthritis, although research in this area is currently lacking.

GUM DISEASE AND BACTERIAL ENDOCARDITIS

Bacterial endocarditis is a heart problem that has often been associated with teeth. Dentists have long been concerned that aggressive bacteria found in periodontal pockets, or the by-products the bacteria trigger, could enter the bloodstream. Particularly in susceptible patients, they could circulate in the body and lodge on roughened blood vessels to form plaque, which could narrow those blood vessels and increase the risk of a clot formation or blockage. If they attached themselves to the lining of the heart or heart valves and multiplied, they could cause the heart muscle or valves to become infected and inflamed.

Once endocarditis is diagnosed, treatment usually consists of intravenous antibiotics. Recovery may take four to six weeks, and there is a risk of permanent heart damage.

Bacterial endocarditis is a real concern for anyone with damaged or artificial heart valves. Consequently, for decades dentists have administered antibiotics immediately before and after cleanings or extractions to people believed to be at risk for this infection.

GUM DISEASE AND PRETERM BIRTHS

Perhaps one of the most fascinating findings from the research connecting dental health with general health is the fact that a relationship has been reported between gum disease and preterm births.[4] In cases where pregnant mothers had healthy gums during pregnancy, researchers found that their babies were more likely to be delivered at full term. Interestingly, women I know who have been using xylitol and the oral care program outlined in this book enjoyed perfect dental health throughout pregnancy and delivered their babies around two weeks later than the normal forty weeks. Several studies show that the more gum disease in a mother's mouth, the greater her chance of delivering her baby early.

In some studies, researchers found that cleaning the mother's mouth during pregnancy could lower this risk, but well-designed studies of recent years have shown that cleanings do not reduce this risk after a woman is pregnant. More research is needed to better understand the situation, but it appears that there may be up to an 84 percent less chance of a premature birth if a mother enters pregnancy with healthy gum conditions.[5] Working to gain a truly healthy mouth is a simple way to help protect your baby from the drastic risks associated with premature birth, which include respiratory problems, long-term disabilities, imperfect organ development, vision impairment, hearing loss, mental retardation, and even death. If you are even thinking about starting a family, you may want to begin a simple home preventive program today to control dental disease in your mouth for your own health, as well as the general health and well-being of your baby.

Preventing Gum Disease

To prevent gum disease, watch for the first signs of infection (bleeding gums) and take action immediately. When you prevent or stop gum disease at the early stage, you avoid all the problems that aggressive periodontal bacteria can inflict on your gums, bones, and health.

Gum disease is rarely seen around baby teeth. The permanent adult teeth start to erupt when a child is around five or six years old. It is important to teach your children the symptoms of gum disease and how to control it during their teen years. The condition of your children's gums can deteriorate quickly as they enter their late teens and early twenties. If you help your children eliminate harmful bacteria from their mouths for a continuous period of two or more years, this positive effect may be long-lived. Steps that you take to improve the health of your children's mouths during childhood can help them control and possibly overcome the challenges of dental disease in early adulthood. Preparing teens for college may now include preparing their mouths in advance of a time when oral hygiene may not be their top priority.

When your teeth have multiple exposures to xylitol each day, totalling at least 6.5 and 10 grams of xylitol, studies show that you can radically change the kind of bacteria in your mouth within one year.[6] (See chapter 12 for a full, detailed discussion about the numerous benefits of consuming xylitol.) This change may have a dramatic effect on the health of your mouth, even for people who cannot or will not floss. More serious types of gum problems may not be resolved with this treatment alone because this will depend on how much damage has already occurred around your teeth and how little bone remains to support them. Gaining control over your oral health will nevertheless be a benefit, and starting the system described in part V will help arrest disease in a simple and easy way.

The next thing to do is visit a dentist as soon as possible to have an evaluation and to learn about remedies that can help return your mouth to health. Gum disease is very destructive and should always be prevented as early as possible, because advanced stages are far more difficult to correct and usually require more radical treatments. Studies indicate that once it has occurred, curing periodontal disease does not guarantee the reversal of the associated general health problems. Therefore, prevention is definitely better than a cure.

Preventing gum infections further helps patients lower their risk for certain health problems and may even help them decrease a need for medications. New studies show that reducing periodontitis may help diabetic patients stabilize insulin levels.[7] As stated earlier in this chapter, it is clear that patients who have such medical problems as diabetes or defective heart valves or who have suffered heart attacks should take preventive dental action quickly to rid their mouths of harmful bacteria and damaging mouth conditions.

PART FOUR

Myths and Truths

With all the scientific evidence that we have about caries prevention, why is it that dental practice has not embraced the concepts of prevention and intervention? It is time for a paradigm shift.

—John Featherstone, M.Sc., Ph.D.

CHAPTER EIGHT

Fluoride

Many people are confused about preventing dental disease and do not realize that damage is most often the end result of a contagious, transmissible infection. The bacteria of this infection weaken teeth and cause gum disease. Harmful bacteria grow and flourish in an acidic or dry mouth and inflict damage to teeth as corrosive acidity weakens tooth enamel to a breaking point.

Preventing this disease is therefore a matter of limiting the bacteria of dental infection and protecting teeth from mouth acidity. Certain mouth cleaning strategies and xylitol are useful for this and will be described in chapters 13 and 14. Another useful prevention method is fortifying normal tooth strength. Constantly building the strength of your teeth helps them to resist acidic damage but it can also rebuild previously weakened teeth. To build the strength of teeth more quickly, xylitol and fluoride can be used together in harmony. This chapter will try to unravel the many viewpoints that surround the controversial topic of fluoride.

The History of Fluoride

Why do we put fluoride into our drinking water? The answer dates to a time when people did not fully understand how fluoride works, how cavities form, or the potential complication of finding that fluoride, or its compounds, reacts with the metals, chemicals, or pharmaceuticals present in modern-day drinking water.

The story of fluoride and dentistry is interesting and remarkable, particularly because it was the harmful effects of fluoride that sparked interest during the early 1900s.[1] Before that time, the only mention of fluoride in dentistry was in records from Europe of calcium fluoride powder being made into a paste to coat teeth in order to strengthen them.

In 1901, a newly graduated American dentist named Frederick McKay noticed that many of his patients' teeth were severely stained brown. McKay worked in Colorado Springs where, with the help of a well-known dental expert, G.V. Black, he investigated samples of these stained teeth under a microscope. The two men noticed gaps in the enamel where it had not formed properly. With their stains and strange defects, these teeth became a topic of discussion among dentists from other parts of the United States and around the world. Many of the doctors had seen similar teeth, and they shared information about them in letters and at meetings.

In all cases, despite the poorly formed enamel with its pitting and staining, the teeth did not appear to develop cavities. In 1923 McKay suspected that the brown stains were caused by something in the water supply that children were drinking. McKay arranged for the water supply line to be changed from its original source, and within ten years, the stained teeth had stopped forming.

By the 1940s almost four hundred areas in twenty-six states had identified teeth with similar brown markings. The U.S. Public Health Service became involved, and an official named H. Trendly Dean was put in charge of the investigation. Dean recorded the severity of the tooth defects he investigated and graded the problems he saw as mild, moderate, or severe. He found a close association between the degree of the mottling and the amount of naturally occurring fluoride in the water. Dean showed that when the amount of fluoride was higher, the mottling on the teeth increased, and when it was less, the mottling was reduced. Because of this association, the enamel condition was called *fluorosis.*

Dean compared the number of cavities he found in teeth with the amount of fluoride in the water in twenty-one American cities and discovered that in areas with a concentration of one to two parts per million of fluoride in the water, cases of moderate and severe fluorosis were rare, but the number of cavities was reduced. Dean was aware that enamel fluorosis occurred in these areas, but he believed that the cosmetic issue was not a problem. Based on his observation, one to two parts per million was adopted as the optimal level for fluoride in our drinking water. During the 1952 Delaney Committee congressional hearings, scientists expressed concern that the dosage was too high, especially for children or people with diabetes or kidney disease, but the ADA endorsed the idea, and adjustments to our water supplies have been made ever since.

A strange connection exists between the Aluminum Company of America (present-day Alcoa) and the fluoridation of water. That aluminum-manufacturing company has always been closely involved in fluoride studies, which is understandable when you know that fluoride is a major waste product of the aluminum industry. During the 1930s and 1940s, this fluoride by-product was used as a registered pesticide in the USA, but more potent chemicals were gradually replacing it in American agriculture. With lack of demand, disposal of fluoride was becoming a problem, at significant cost to the industry. At the same time, the American economy was struggling, and records show that aluminum company engineers were energetically looking for new markets and ways to improve sales. Many fingers have been pointed at the politics and people involved in the original fluoride decision-making process, the scathing critiques of the initial study designs, and the reporting of the results.

Pros and Cons of Using Fluoride

The fluoride debate begun in the 1930s has continued ever since, both inside and outside the dental profession. On one extreme there are citizen groups vehemently opposed to public water fluoridation who raise serious questions and valid concerns, but on the other side there are those who beat the drum for fluoride, often unaware of the dubious parts to the story and good alternative approaches that are available. Today many well-respected dentists, physicians, and researchers voice opposition to fluoridation and ask to study more closely the effect that this chemical is having on residential water supplies.[2] Although health concerns include almost everything, of particular concern are neurological problems, reduced intelligence, and certain forms of cancer.

Arguments against water fluoridation become stronger when products like xylitol are shown to easily and effectively control tooth decay. In Switzerland, salt is a medium for fluroide; consumers have the choice of fluoridated or non-fluoridated salt. Milk fluoridation is another idea, implemented in parts of Eastern Europe, China, and South America. Milk that is fluoridated could be used in school-based programs, particularly for high-risk populations. The cost of such programs would be smaller, and the method possibly more appropriate than water fluoridation.

In 1999, the U.S. Environmental Protection Agency (EPA) reviewed studies from Binghamton University in New York. The scientists had reported kidney and brain damage in rats exposed to half the amount of fluoride added to our water supplies. The National Toxicology Program conducted further studies in conjunction with Procter & Gamble to determine the extent of neurotoxic damage, particularly stressing fluoride's interaction with aluminum.

Although the results were negative, many people continue to be skeptical, citing too close an association between Alcoa and Procter & Gamble. In fact, an entire book has been written describing the special interests of these companies, the historical sequence of events, and possible links between fluoride and the Manhattan Project of World War II.[3]

ALUMINUM AND FLUORIDE

There has been a great deal of conversation in the dental world about claims that fluoride has a strong affinity for aluminum. Since the 1990s, there have been concerns that aluminum and fluoride together could be responsible for the alarming increase in Alzheimer's disease and senile dementia.[4] Officials in the ADA department responsible for water fluoridation assure me that the official word from the Alzheimer's association is that no connection between Alzheimer's and fluoride has ever been found.

In 1987 the Medical Research Endocrinology Department at Newcastle upon Tyne, England, performed experiments where fluoridated water (one part per million) was boiled in an aluminum pan. The studies showed that when fluoride was in the water, aluminum leached out of the pan. The boiling fluoridated tap water leached almost 200 parts per million of aluminum from the aluminum pan into the water in ten minutes, and up to 600 parts per million with prolonged boiling. Varying amounts of aluminum were released depending on the type of pan and depending on the variety of foods cooked in the pan.

The more acidic the liquid, the more aluminum leached. Using non-fluoridated water showed almost no leaching from aluminum pans.

When water supplies are from surface water, the treatment facilities routinely add aluminum sulphate prior to the water fluoridation process to remove sediment. In 2000 the National Institute of Environmental Health Sciences acknowledged that fluoride can increase the uptake of aluminum in water, depending on the acidity of the water (that is, its pH). There are reports, most somewhat difficult to substantiate, that claim fluoride may interact with substances in water and create the potential for toxic fluoro-aluminum compounds to form. Officials dispute such claims.

If the combination of aluminum and fluoride worries you, another cause for concern should be the amount of aluminum contained in consumable products, from soy formula to dried infant formulas. Infant formula can contain up to sixty-three times more aluminum than breast milk, and there may be cause for concern about mixing this formula powder with fluoridated water. Baking soda, many processed foods, frozen dough, and even tea may contain varying amounts of aluminum. Nondairy creamer (94 parts per million), Oreo cookies (127 parts per million), antacid medications, and buffered aspirin also have high levels of aluminum. Drinks and foods may be stored in aluminum cans, and many soft drinks are made with fluoridated water. Perhaps someone should take an unopened soda that is a few years old and have a laboratory analyze the ingredients!

Today the majority of people are ingesting fluoride from so many different sources, they are receiving far in excess of the amount originally intended.[5] These problems, combined with a new understanding of how fluoride works, have created confusion and again fueled the debate about whether or not fluoride is healthy for you and your family. I believe that water supplies, particularly in areas where aluminum sulphate is added, should be studied closely and staunch advocates should take a second look from an evidence-based perspective at the studies from which fluoridation decisions were made. Clear impartial evaluation is the only way to answer legitimate concerns that many have voiced about the quality of our drinking water in the United States.

After sixty years, it may be time to revisit the issue of water fluoridation. We must realize that fluoridation of water is not a miracle cure for teeth and that it may have possible drawbacks that were not foreseen at the start. The overriding problem of adding fluoride to municipal drinking water appears to be the potential of ingesting too much and the negative impact on our health of its interaction with such metals as aluminum and lead. Questionable studies, heavy-handed dismissal of dissenters, and a strange aura surround water fluoridation and certainly give cause for concern.

Fluoride Misconceptions

A number of people with "soft teeth" worry that their problems have been caused by a lack of fluoride in their drinking water. These people often complain that their water supplies have been neglected by those responsible for public health. They mistakenly assume that fluoride benefits teeth as a vitamin might benefit overall health. On the other hand, some people fear fluoride so much that they refuse to even rinse with it. A number of people, unfortunately, will even go as far as to permit tooth damage—to the point of needing a filling, crown, or extraction—rather than put any kind of fluoride in their mouths.

I straddle the fluoride argument. I see benefits from a good fluoride mouth rinse and fluoride in toothpaste, but I am not an advocate for adding it to our drinking water. Water without fluoride will never be the cause of weak or soft teeth. As you have learned, mouth acidity creates tooth softening that leads to cavities and dental problems.

I have weighed any negative facts about fluoride with the positive outcomes it can produce. I have looked at the teeth of those who will not use fluoride in any form and compared them with those who follow my oral care recommendations. The differences in dental health are quite remarkable. Some people fear that fluoride may be absorbed through the skin during rinsing. There is no evidence to substantiate these worries, and I believe that any minuscule risk would be dwarfed by the numerous health benefits that strong and unfilled teeth offer us.

Suppose you have damaged your teeth in some way, for example by drinking soda. Under healthy mouth conditions, the rebuilding of tooth enamel will occur naturally, but if fluoride is involved in the process, these repairs occur more quickly, and the new enamel will be stronger. Fluoride plays its part by stimulating teeth to rebuild themselves after they have become damaged. Fluoride works as an instigator or catalyst to speed up the process of natural tooth remineralization that repairs weak teeth. Remember, it was the soda that caused the damage to the tooth, not a lack of fluoride.

Used correctly, fluoride can help both children and adults avoid fillings and keep their teeth healthy for life. For tooth health, it appears that fluoride does not need to be ingested, used as a consumable supplement, or applied as a high-concentration gel.

As a matter of fact, when fluoride is ingested, around 93 percent is absorbed and flows around your body in the bloodstream. The kidneys in a healthy individual excrete most of the fluoride, but any that remains in the body is permanently deposited into the skeleton. Thus, the efficiency of the kidneys is vital, because kidney function affects the amount of fluoride that remains in your body. Kidney disease lowers the efficiency of fluoride elimination, and people with kidney problems should always use non-fluoridated water.

We used to think that fluoride was inactivated in milk, but that is not correct. The topical effect of fluoride on teeth remains the same whether it is in water or in milk. The difference is that when it is consumed in milk, or with calcium-rich foods, less fluoride will be absorbed into the bloodstream. This useful effect of combining calcium with fluoride lowers the amount of fluoride absorbed from 93 percent to about 60 percent, which explains why anyone who accidentally ingests too much fluoride is usually given milk to drink.

In my own dental practice in England, I noticed both benefits and problems with fluoride as I looked at the teeth of my family, friends, and patients. Later in my career I revisited the subject of fluoride during my graduate studies in the USA. It was interesting to examine in close detail the questions and concerns I had noted over the years. Since that time I have unearthed many surprising facts about fluoride that make up a complicated story about its use for dental health.

Today I use a professionally installed fluoride filter to purify the drinking water in my home. I teach my patients that the strengthening effect of fluoride on teeth is mainly topical, so there is no need to drink or consume fluoride to have nice teeth. In fact, ingesting too much fluoride may not only be damaging to your health but can be especially harmful to developing enamel.

Sources of Fluoride

Fluoride is carried into our homes from many sources besides drinking water. It can be found in manufactured foods, sodas, beer, infant formula, and powdered iced tea (go to www.cleanwhiteteeth.com for a list of fluoride content in foods). Your personal daily consumption of fluoride from tap water depends on how much liquid you consume each day (including soups, coffee or tea, other liquids, and cooked products). Obviously if you are athletic and live in a warm climate, you will drink far more water than someone sedentary who lives in a colder climate. A one-size-fits-all approach does not seem appropriate for gauging a safe fluoride dose from drinking water, and it may be that some people are consuming too much fluoride from this source.

The EPA sets the standard for fluoride in community drinking water, and 62.2 percent of water supplies in the USA today are fluoridated. As a result, about 160 million people in the United States drink artificially fluoridated water. The ADA also passionately supports fluoridation. Fluoride cannot be removed from drinking water with a charcoal filter, and for many years the reverse-osmosis filter or steam distilling process was the only way to remove it. Now, however, there are various filter systems capable of removing fluoride from your home water supply. Many websites post information about fluoride-filtration systems, or you could consult a local water filtration expert in your area.[6] One word of caution: Distilled water may be chemically pure, but because it is devoid of all minerals, it often can have an aggressive effect on dental enamel.

Yet another factor to consider with regard to fluoridation is the *halo effect*. This refers to the spreading of fluoride from one geographic area to another when beverages, foods, and other fluoride-containing products are produced in one area to be consumed elsewhere.

By means of the halo effect, most people in the United States receive fluoride by consuming products that have been manufactured in fluoridated areas. Studies during the 1940s showed only 15 percent of teeth with mild fluorosis; moderate or severe forms were rare. Forty years later, mild fluorosis was seen in almost 25 percent of teeth, and a small percentage of teeth showed moderate or severe forms of fluorosis.[7] Today these figures are much higher, and fluorosis is seen everywhere, even in geographic areas with low-fluoride and non-fluoride water.

Sodium Fluoride

When people say fluoride has been added to their water, they really mean that a fluoride compound has been added. Mouth rinses and toothpastes contain various kinds of fluoride. For example, Crest Regular paste contains sodium fluoride, whereas the newer Crest Pro-Health contains *stannous fluoride*, a compound derived from tin. (Stannous fluoride was popular in the 1960s because it was shown to reduce gum inflammation. The problem with stannous fluoride, however, is that it creates unattractive black or brown staining on teeth.) The addition of minerals to fluoride rinses does not increase its effectiveness for people with normal saliva, but the extra ingredients usually make it more expensive than other fluoride rinses.

I recommend only sodium fluoride, which has been studied for decades and is the most stable and safe. And it will not stain teeth, a problem that can occur with other kinds of fluoride, particularly stannous fluoride.

Unfortunately, sodium fluoride is the most expensive fluoride, so it is rarely used for fluoridation of our water supplies. More than 90 percent of the fluoridated water in the United States comes from a silicofluoride (either fluorosilicic acid or sodium silicofluoride). These chemicals differ from the simpler sodium fluoride in many ways and may react differently with other chemicals. Many people are concerned that silicofluorides increase the uptake of lead in the body, which could ironically generate higher rates of tooth decay and a host of other problems, including learning disabilities and attention deficit disorder. The ADA spokesperson denies that such reactions are possible, but perhaps more research would allay public worries and fears.

Fluoride Mouth Rinse

I am completely convinced about the positive effects seen in the teeth of those who regularly use a dilute sodium fluoride mouth rinse. A final rinse each night and a first rinse each morning appear to protect and beautify teeth for patients of all ages. Many people think fluoride will help only children's teeth, and they are shocked to find that its protective effects are just as useful for the teeth of people in their eighties as they are for those in their teens.

Perhaps, like me, you grind your teeth. Without extra-strong teeth, I would most certainly have damaged my teeth by now, possibly causing old fillings to loosen or pieces of enamel to chip away and break off. To give my teeth extra strength and resist tooth damage, I use a dilute fluoride rinse in my oral care routine every morning and every night.

Years ago we believed that the benefits of fluoride were built into teeth before they erupted into the mouth. Today we know that fluoride mainly benefits teeth when it is in direct contact with the outside tooth surface. The benefit ends as soon as fluoride is washed away. To strengthen a tooth, fluoride needs to bathe the outside for as long as possible. Fluoride rebuilds teeth by helping to move minerals from saliva into areas of weak or damaged tooth enamel. The longer the contact time between fluoride and the tooth, the more minerals will go into the enamel to harden teeth.

Any tooth enamel that repairs in the presence of fluoride has a particle of fluoride included in its structure. This small change to the chemistry of the enamel makes the tooth surface become stronger, smoother, and more acid resistant than before. From a patient's point of view this makes the outside of a tooth extra strong and shiny and less able to be damaged by acidity in the future.

I advise patients to avoid high-concentration fluoride products and look for lower-dilution products, such as ACT, with 0.05 percent fluoride, which, ironically, can be more effective in strengthening your teeth than gels and pastes that contain ten times the concentration of fluoride. A recent evidence-based review of topical fluoride products showed that very strong gels and foams (the kind used in dental offices for treating children's teeth) may have little or no effect on strengthening the teeth of children who already have good teeth.[8]

My patients with the healthiest teeth usually rinse with ACT, which comes in mint, cinnamon, and bubble-gum flavors. A new ACT has been produced with "freshening" additives, but it contains ingredients that appear to alter its effectiveness. Large stores make their own formulation of the rinse as a generic product, but those rinses appear to be less effective than the original. Whatever kind of fluoride rinse you choose, I suggest you find one that does not include alcohol. Finding ACT in some parts of the United States and Europe has proven to be a problem, but Internet ordering can help.

Weak and strong fluorides work differently. This may be one reason why a dilute fluoride may work to strengthen your child's teeth more than a stronger one. A weak fluoride works as a catalyst, helping build minerals into teeth—as described earlier—whereas a strong fluoride gel works by inactivating bacterial enzymes, temporarily stopping the bacteria from producing the acids that damage teeth.

Interestingly, the volume or amount of fluoride that bathes your tooth is of no importance. A few drops of a fluoride mouth rinse will work just as well as a large mouthful. The manufacturers of mouth rinse would like you to use as much as possible, but the truth is, you can be economical with your rinse and still do a complete job. Try to keep fluoride in contact with your tooth surfaces for as long as possible; the longer the duration of contact, the stronger your tooth enamel will become.

Adults (and children with adult teeth) will benefit from using a dilute 0.05 percent sodium fluoride rinse without alcohol the last thing before going to bed. If you rinse and spit out but do not wash your mouth or drink anything more, a thin residue will cover your teeth for many hours during the night. The residue helps minerals in saliva rebuild damaged tooth enamel to improve the condition of your teeth while you are sleeping. The treatment will be especially helpful for people with tooth damage caused by dry mouth, acid reflux, or trauma to teeth from a hard bite.

The more often you rinse with fluoride, the more help you give your teeth; there does not seem to be any amount of time that is too short to provide some benefit. Rinsing several times a day will speed and improve results if you are trying to strengthen your teeth or repair damage. Fluoride as a liquid rinse enters the small crevices and grooves in teeth, even under and around braces or bridgework, to strengthen places that are often the most inaccessible to a toothbrush and at greatest risk for cavities.

If a fluoride rinse is used regularly, it constantly rebuilds the strength of teeth and prevents weakness, sensitivity, and cavities from forming. Fluoride rinsing offers insurance against progressive damage to your teeth. If you dislike or fear dental treatments or are concerned about the health-related problems of filling materials, fluoride rinsing should be your lifelong friend!

Children's Teeth and Fluoride

Fluoride is especially important as teeth emerge into the mouth of a young child. Permanent teeth come into the mouth in a sequence, normally starting with four back-molar teeth. Adults with otherwise good teeth frequently have cavities in these first permanent molars, found about halfway along the jaw, both upper and lower, on the side of the mouth. First permanent molars erupt around kindergarten or first grade, behind the row of baby teeth and usually before any sign of a loose tooth.

First permanent molars have a high rate of decay, often forming cavities within a year of their eruption. It has been estimated that 70 to 93 percent of first permanent molars have tooth damage within two years of erupting, and most of the damage occurs within the first twelve months. Pediatric dentists are accustomed to seeing children who, before their teeth have even had time to harden, need crowns, root-canal treatments, or even extraction.

Fluoride speeds up the absorption of minerals by enamel, and in this way it can shorten the time of hardening or maturation that occurs as a tooth erupts into the mouth. Fluoride rinsing can speed this maturation process and increase the odds that a child's new tooth will remain cavity free for life. Twelve-year molars and wisdom teeth are just as vulnerable when they erupt, entering a teenager's mouth with compromised protection. These molars are normally the last teeth to erupt, and they frequently cause problems because they are at the back of the mouth and difficult to clean.

New front teeth that erupt at around seven or eight years of age are also soft as they enter the mouth. Soft teeth usually look dark or yellowish in color. There is nothing wrong with these teeth, and with sufficient time they will harden and lighten in color. Any bleaching of these newly erupted teeth can seriously weaken an already weak tooth; therefore, it is not recommended. It is much safer to help new teeth harden and mature as quickly as possible by rinsing with a dilute fluoride rinse and eating xylitol. Both these products have been shown to assist and encourage mineralization of the outer shell of tooth enamel, which will make teeth stronger and appear whiter quickly, often within a year.

Maturation is dramatically slowed in the mouth of a child with a blocked nose, asthma, or allergies or for any child taking mouth-drying medications. The mineralizing process is less complete for children with acidic mouths from acid reflux, poor diets, or chronic illness. Cavities and worn-down teeth will cause such children discomfort, dental pain, and the need for fillings and crowns even before first grade. Mineralization, on the other hand, is more efficient in the alkaline mouth of a healthy child. In all circumstances, maturation is encouraged and enhanced with the use of a fluoride rinse and xylitol together in a program of preventive oral care.

Fluoride is not a vitamin. If babies consume a fraction too much fluoride before the age of three, it may poison the cells that form healthy tooth enamel. *Ameloblasts* are the enamel-forming cells found in the jaws of infants and babies, and they are the cells that produce the materials that develop into the outer enamel of our teeth. Ameloblasts are very sensitive and are easily poisoned by fluoride. If these cells die, the teeth still grow, but gaps occur where the enamel does not form properly. Such enamel defects are seen on teeth as white or (in more severe cases) brown spots and is the condition known as fluorosis.

Human breast milk has a very low fluoride concentration, regardless of the mother's intake. Commercially prepared formula, on the other hand, can have very high fluoride levels. Manufacturers have been told to reduce the amount of fluoride in their formula milk and baby-food concentrates following a study in Iowa of dried infant milk.[9] The study showed that the babies were consuming too much fluoride and in erratic amounts from formula products. The study showed that the fluoride in infant formula could cause fluorosis of varying degrees, especially in cases where the powdered formula was reconstituted with fluoridated tap water. (Note: If a meal is prepared with fluoridated water that has been boiled for some time, steam will evaporate away a percentage of the water and leave the remaining liquid with an increased concentration of fluoride in it.)

My five children were born between 1977 and 1990. I gave my first child fluoride drops in the recommended concentration because I lived in an area without fluoride in the water. At that time dentists believed that giving fluoride drops to infants would work internally to make their teeth grow more perfectly, with smoother surfaces and more resistance to decay. My first daughter was born in 1977, and it was not until her two permanent front teeth erupted when she was eight years old that I discovered they had been changed by this fluoride; there were brown defects in the center of each one. Her enamel-forming cells had been poisoned by the five fluoride drops I conscientiously added to her drinks each day when she was a baby. Such defects in teeth are given the name *moderate fluorosis*, and to correct their appearance would require cosmetic dental repair with crowns or veneers to mask the damage.

I gave less fluoride to my second daughter, who was born in 1980, because dosage recommendations had changed and because I was a busy mother. She now has small cloud-like spots over her permanent front and side teeth, a condition of mild fluorosis and the result of similar but slightly less poisoning of her enamel-producing cells. My other children have never received fluoride supplements, and we now filter fluoride out of our drinking water at home. On the other hand, since the age of about six (when they could rinse and spit), all my children have used a dilute fluoride rinse twice a day. My younger children's teeth are beautiful and without defects.

Some physicians and dentists still prescribe fluoride tablets to children, and the discussion continues between dentists and doctors, some believing that fluoride's protection occurs from the inside of the tooth while others, like myself, prefer to rely on the benefits that fluoride provides directly to the surface of teeth. Parents should know that the Academy of Pediatric Dentistry suggests that children under three, who are prone to eating toothpaste, should not use any fluoride-containing paste.

If you have cavities but do not want to go to a dentist, fluoride rinsing, especially combined with the use of xylitol, will help stop their progression. If you use fluoridated toothpaste, you can make a less-expensive mouth rinse from toothpaste mixed with water. I recommend original Crest toothpaste that contains sodium fluoride. Make sure it is a paste without plaque control or whitening additives, which have unnecessary chemicals in them and can be abrasive. Use the normal amount of toothpaste on your brush and clean your teeth in the usual way. Before spitting out, sip a small amount of water (about a tablespoon) and swish the water around your teeth, creating a dilute sodium fluoride rinse in the concentration that works to harden teeth.

Only children who can safely spit should use a fluoride rinse. If your child needs the healing help of fluoride for damaged teeth, I recommend brushing a young child's teeth with a drop of ACT on the toothbrush in place of toothpaste. We are not looking for children to drink fluoride, so experiment with your children using plain water to determine if they can achieve the rinsing and spitting maneuver safely before you give them a fluoride rinse. I encourage parents to slowly add drops of the fluoride rinse to the water as the child's ability improves, until finally the child will be using a full-strength and undiluted rinse.

Most of us need to spit twice (one spit followed immediately by another spit) to effectively remove the rinse from our mouths. Encourage young children to spit one more time, because extra spitting is fun for them and ensures that they do not hold extra rinse in their mouths and swallow it. Do not use any other rinse, and avoid drinking after your fluoride rinse, because you want to leave a microscopic film of it on your teeth to protect them during the night.

Dentist-Applied Fluoride Treatments

The amount of fluoride in a liquid, food, or product is measured in parts per million. Water supplies are fluoridated to a designated "optimal" level of between one and two parts per million. Fluoride gels and foams that dentists use in their offices usually have concentrations of fluoride between 9,000 and 12,300 parts per million, and most of them are so strongly acidic that the products could easily etch the surface of a porcelain sink. In May 2006 the ADA's Council of Scientific Affairs published a report about the effectiveness of fluoride treatments, using an evidence-based method. The results were surprising to many dentists because they showed that, especially for decay-free children, fluoride gels and foams are not considered clinically relevant, because there is *no measurable benefit from applying them to healthy teeth*. Only when fluoride gels were used for a minimum of four minutes did they appear to help children with active disease (new cavities) or serious tooth decay and to help harden newly erupted molar teeth. One-minute applications of fluoride foam were a quick and convenient treatment in the 1990s, but they have been shown to be ineffective.[10] Results show that stronger fluoride works to kill bacteria but is less effective in strengthening teeth, so new recommendations for strengthening teeth advocate frequent exposure to low-dose fluoride.

FLUORIDE VARNISH

The data from the ADA's evidence-based review of the studies showed that the best results from dentist-applied fluoride treatment were repeatedly found with fluoride varnish for children of all ages who are at risk for cavities. This treatment has been used in preventive programs in Europe for more than thirty years. The varnish is a sticky mixture that dries onto teeth and slowly gives out low doses of fluoride over weeks and often months, finally wearing itself away. It is an exciting option, especially for special-needs and noncompliant children and those who are sick or at some special risk for cavities. Applying fluoride varnish is simple and painless for the child, takes less time for the dentist, and requires no tooth preparation. The best news is the overall protection this treatment offers to baby and permanent teeth. The evidence-based review showed that for patients at high risk, fluoride varnish applied twice a year gave "significant help to prevent cavities."[11]

When fluoride varnishes first appeared on the market, their worst feature was their unattractive yellow color, but today they are colorless. If any tooth has poorly formed enamel or a soft spot, fluoride varnish can offer preventive help. Fluoride varnish applied to newly erupted teeth, combined with consumption of xylitol, seems like an ideal treatment, since it helps prevent cavities and may speed up tooth maturation, so these new teeth gain their natural and unique protective covering more quickly.

Most dentists have trouble digesting the various arguments about fluoride, but it becomes more confusing to see the logo of the American Academy of Pediatric Dentistry on the Coca-Cola product called Spring Water and advertised as "Fluoride to Go." The academy says that the logo does not imply endorsement of the bottled water, which contains added fluoride, but most mothers would assume the product is healthy and beneficial for children.

In a perfect world, where acidic liquids never touch teeth and we never age or have acidic, dry mouths, fluoride would be unnecessary. In real life many foods, drinks, medications, and conditions beyond our control are risk factors that put us in need of extra help. This is where the latest evidence shows fluoride to be a useful tool, especially when used as a low-dose rinse or a varnish to help reduce the need for fillings and dental treatments. At the very least, fluoridated water may provide the public with a free mouth rinse to swish around teeth after meals as protection against cavities. Whether you should drink this water or not is a subject for another book.

CHAPTER NINE

Sealants

In the early 1980s new techniques for adhering fillings to teeth were developed. It was exciting to find a method that allowed a filling to glue itself onto the surface of a tooth without the need for cutting down the tooth.

Preparing a tooth for a filling in the old days meant making cuts and grooves to help the tooth retain the filling. This new technique instead involves etching the tooth and filling the micropores that open up with a plastic resin. This technique was particularly useful for very small fillings and to fill in pits in a tooth surface. Finally, it became a means to obliterate grooves in molar teeth. By doing this, a dentist is able to prevent bacteria from breeding in the grooves of a child's molar teeth, the places which provide reservoirs of bacteria for the mouth. This kind of filling is called a *sealant* because it is able to seal tooth grooves.

Today dentists often suggest placing a sealant in a child's new tooth. The idea is to protect the tooth and remove the space that normally provides refuge to acid-producing bacteria. The process that a dentist will use involves cleaning the tooth and keeping it dry long enough to squirt plastic material into the groove and harden it up, often under a strong light source.

Sealants became more generally used during the early 1990s, and at first glance they seem to be a terrific idea. The process appears simple, and as long as the sealant remains in place, mouth liquids and bacteria will not be able to enter tooth grooves, and this will prevent cavities from forming. The story is not quite so simple, however, and there are a number of things that everyone agreeing to a sealant should understand. There are certainly situations where sealants have value, but there are a number of issues to consider first.

A cause for concern involves the fact that sealants may release a substance called bisphenol A, recently found to leach out of baby bottle plastics. Bisphenol A can mimic estrogen and, although this was disputed in the past, new research shows that small amounts may be more damaging to health than larger amounts. ADA information on this subject has been upgraded recently and consumer fears have been calmed. Nevertheless I believe some concern exists and, since dental materials vary, ramifications should be discussed with your dentist before agreeing to sealant placement.

Sealants can be a barrier only if they remain in place. The success or failure of sealants is therefore determined by how long the sealant lasts. Sealants are never expected to stay in place for more than a few years, and so they must be reapplied. Today, even in the best conditions, about 10 percent of sealants fail within twelve months of being put on teeth.[1] Research in 2000 showed that when a sealant is lost, the uncovered area of the tooth will once again be at risk of becoming a cavity.[2]

Sealants and Bacteria

A number of dentists share the concern that a sealant could be sealing over the top of bacteria, leaving some trapped inside these grooves. A special technique was devised to clean the groove before sealing it. A dental cutting instrument was developed for this cleaning process, one similar to the instruments, called *burs*, used to cut away a tooth for a filling. The irony of this is that the tooth now has a mini-cavity to protect it from a cavity!

Evidence-based research is a method of looking at many studies and evaluating the results under stringent scientific standards, so as to have the most accurate and unbiased information available. The National Institutes of Health and the ADA have evaluated many preventive treatment methods so as to guide dentists in their clinical decisions. When sealants were reviewed using this evidence-based method, the results showed that nothing bad will happen if bacteria mistakenly become trapped under a sealant—provided that they have no contact with the outside world. If bacteria are cut off from their food supply, they will just lie quietly without causing damage. The problem is that there are many brands of sealant, and we do not know if they are all equally efficient at sealing teeth.[3] Most dentists worry that if a sealant breaks down, liquids could seep underneath and reconnect bacteria with the outside world. For this reason, once a sealant has been placed, it will need to be checked every six months for the rest of your child's life or until it falls off! If it is not checked, there is the risk that the sealant can become a hazard and actually help create a cavity. Once a tooth has a sealant in it, it is no longer a pristine tooth; it is, rather, one that will need constant supervision.

Although harmful bacteria may have been blocked by a sealant from entering a molar groove, these bacteria of dental disease will continue to be present elsewhere in the mouth. Sealants do little to decrease the general population of harmful bacteria in the mouth or teach a patient about the ongoing risk factors. The biting surfaces of molars may be blocked, but other surfaces of the teeth will continue to be attacked until they weaken, become damaged, and form cavities, most often at vulnerable areas where teeth contact other teeth. The surfaces that touch each other are called *interproximal areas,* and cavities are often found on X-rays about three to five years after the initial sealants were applied to the biting surface grooves. The reality is that there is no way for a sealant to protect the sides of the teeth, and there is no way for sealants to stop interproximal cavities from forming.

Sealants for Children

Although sealants offer temporary protection to the most vulnerable biting surfaces in the mouth, parents need to realize the limitations of sealants and know about the available alternatives. Studies have shown that sealants can lower molar decay rates by up to 76.3 percent after four years, provided they are checked and reapplied whenever they are chipped or broken. On the other hand, a study in 2000 compared school-age children who chewed xylitol gum regularly with children treated with professionally applied sealants. After five years there was no difference between the groups. The protection offered by chewing xylitol gum was equal to that offered by a sealant.[4]

The most logical plan, however, is to work to eliminate harmful bacteria from the mouth, with or without sealants. Bacterial cleaning of the mouth is especially important before new molars erupt, no matter whether it is the baby molar of a two-year-old, the first permanent molar of a six-year-old, or a third molar of a twenty-year-old. Fighting to eliminate harmful germs should be everyone's priority, but especially in the year before new teeth are expected (go to www. cleanwhiteteeth.com to see the chart of eruption times for teeth). The greatest concern is for the children at high risk for cavities because of a dry or acidic mouth. This includes almost all children at some time in their childhood, since the list covers those who have acidic saliva, acid reflux, or an active lifestyle, as well as those who enjoy acidic drinks, citrus fruits, or sugary or starchy foods, or who take medications—especially those for allergies or asthma.

Xylitol or Sealants?

One day a friend told me about his teenage son's visit to the dentist. The dentist had found tooth decay in the boy's new molars. The dentist suggested putting sealants on the teeth to prevent the early cavities from growing bigger. He insisted that without sealants the teeth would end up with big cavities by the time of the boy's six-month checkup.

My friend and I had talked about the options with the risks and benefits of sealants, as well as the things his son could do to avoid them. He decided to postpone his son's sealant appointment and instead to use a regimen of fluoride mouth rinsing and mints made with 100 percent xylitol. The boy closely followed the daily regimen for six months; then he went for his next dental checkup. Understandably nervous, the father watched while the dentist checked his son's previously decayed teeth. The dentist looked at his notes and examined the boy's mouth. He looked closely at the molars where cavities had been starting six months previously. The dentist checked the teeth with an explorer. He checked them again, searching for the cavities. The dentist was puzzled to see that the teeth were strong and firm. The teeth had rebuilt themselves, and the cavities were no longer there.

The dentist called his assistant over, insisting that she had forgotten to write in the notes that the sealants had been applied at the previous appointment.

"No sealants were applied," said the father, explaining how he had canceled the appointment. He further explained how the teeth must have repaired themselves with the mouth rinses and xylitol the boy had used. The dentist may have been confused, but my friend was convinced, and he continues to make sure that his son protects his teeth every day with this regimen.

Discuss sealants with your dentist, because they are not the only option for dental health. There is no reason why a groove in a molar tooth cannot remain healthy. The most vulnerable time for this groove is as it erupts into the mouth. Creating a healthy environment for a tooth before it erupts into the mouth is of vital importance. Remember that molar grooves take up to a year to fully harden and that it is acidic attacks that destroy the teeth of teenagers and young adults.

A fluoride varnish is another good preventive method and another alternative to sealants if your child appears to be slightly at risk for cavities. (I discussed this technique in greater detail in chapter 8.) This product sticks in the grooves for several months, helping the tooth to naturally mature and harden its enamel coating. Once the grooves have hardened, they will be better able to resist acid attacks.

Another option for children who are able to safely rinse and spit is twice-daily use of a dilute fluoride rinse, which works in harmony with xylitol and can help to give new adult teeth strength and resistance.

Unfortunately, in many situations sealants are placed on teeth as a routine when they erupt into the mouth. Before you agree to have sealants put on your child's teeth, you may want to think about these alternative ways to protect teeth—ways that enhance natural protection and ultimately leave a natural, pristine tooth in your child's mouth.

CHAPTER TEN

Whitening

If you are going to bleach your teeth, understand what you are doing and evaluate the risks. Today everyone—even small children—wants whiter teeth. In fact, the American Academy of Pediatric Dentistry has recognized a demand for whitening children's teeth and issued new policies about this kind of treatment.[1] During bleaching you can upset or kill the nerve of a tooth, which could potentially require a root-canal treatment or even an extraction. Advertisements by oral care companies appeal to people's desire to improve their teeth, but it is important to understand the difference between white teeth and healthy teeth. Appearances can be deceptive!

Cosmetic Dental Makeovers

Young people today have watched movie stars and celebrities have instant cosmetic makeovers. TV programs give the impression that it is easy to go to a dentist and get a fabulous new smile. People talk about tooth veneers to change the shape, character, and color of teeth in a matter of one or two visits. People who think they inherited bad teeth imagine that a beautiful smile can be purchased like a new outfit for their wardrobe.

Dentists want you to take pride in your teeth. Everyone feels better when their teeth are whiter and their smile is brighter. The problem is that while cosmetic dental makeovers change the shape and color of a smile, they do nothing to address the cause of the problems that disfigured the original teeth, the attack of dental disease. If dental disease caused your problems in the first place, unless you work to change the conditions in your mouth, this disease will continue to attack your teeth, around the margins where false crowns join natural roots, after your makeover.

Individuals with new smiles can find themselves battling receding gums, cavities under the crowns, sensitive teeth, root decay, the need for repairs, and worse. Dental disease may be delayed for a year or two, but a crown, bleaching, or a makeover will not end it. Some people are dismayed to find their makeover treatments need repair after just a couple of years. Only an effective program to change the bacteria in your mouth will keep your teeth healthy and safe for years, possibly forever.

The oral care industry blossomed in the early 1990s and flooded the market with new toothpastes, breath fresheners, stain-removal systems, and finally, whitening products. People—especially teens and young adults—from all walks of life now want to improve the look of their teeth. No longer are white teeth just for movie stars. People without dental insurance think that the over-the-counter products in drugstores will give them a chance to improve and brighten their smiles. There appear to be many choices to whiten your teeth, at every price level.

The public's interest has generated great profits for the major oral care companies over the past twenty years. Sales of whitening products have increased each year, and they doubled between 2000 and 2006. Despite the huge growth in sales, few studies have been done to evaluate the safety of bleaching, especially for the younger teeth of teens or small children. In fact, the only negative study results appear to have been generated in countries outside the United States, or they were published before the oral care industry began to boom.

Marketing campaigns and an overwhelming selection of new products confuse the public. There is a big difference between healthy white teeth and overbleached ones. For many, the interest in whitening teeth has evolved into a near obsession beyond the boundaries of common sense. Recent articles in the *Journal of Pediatric Dentistry* talk of mothers who are bleaching baby teeth.[2] In one study, many children—some as young as ten—wore tooth whitener strips to school each morning.[3] The concern is the lack of research to ensure that there are no detrimental effects from bleaching. Studies have been conducted on adult teeth with mixed results, but baby teeth have thinner protective shells and a bigger pulp inside which contains essential cells, nerves, and blood vessels.

Enamel and Dentin

Everyone should realize that whatever you use to bleach your teeth, you are trying to achieve a *"less-hazardous* effect on the enamel's mineral content." Everyone who bleaches their teeth will damage their enamel to some extent. The problem is that tooth enamel is delicate, and most people do not treat it with the respect it both needs and deserves.

Let's review the important facts about enamel from previous chapters. When your enamel is healthy, it is made up of perfect crystals tightly packed together, making it solid, smooth, and strong. The density of enamel depends on how tightly the crystals are packed, which depends on the quantity of minerals it contains.

Dentin is the tooth layer underneath enamel. It is softer than enamel, has a creamy white color, and is very porous. When you look at dentin under a microscope, you see small tubes radiating from the center of the tooth, through the layer, to the enamel on the outside. At the very center of the tooth, encased by dentin, is the blood supply to the tooth, nerves, and many cells. This is the tooth pulp. If you fracture a tooth and expose the pulp, it will cause bleeding and will expose live nerves. Live cells called *odontoblasts* live underneath the entrance to each of these dentin tubes and these cells continue throughout a tooth's life to build the dentin layer. These cells have extension arms that travel up the inside of the dentin tubes, looking like a Gumby arm stretching out from the cell inside the pulp area. Any change in pressure is transmitted through these cells to the nerve inside the tooth, which is why you feel pain and sensitivity when a dentist cuts or touches the dentin layer with dental instruments.

Many people are surprised to find out that the outside layer of every healthy tooth is colorless—the color of glass—and translucent. When light shines on a tooth it either reflects off the surface or travels through the enamel, reflecting to some extent the color of the dentin layer underneath it. A tooth's whiteness is basically determined by how much light is reflected off the outer surface. If the light is absorbed by a soft enamel surface it will look the color of the dentin underneath—usually a yellowish color.

Variations in how naturally white a tooth appears are therefore determined by the strength of the outer layer. Hard, strong, healthy enamel will behave like a diamond and bounce light off its surface in a way that makes teeth seem brighter and appear whiter, no matter the color of the dentin in the underlying tooth. Soft teeth behave in the opposite way; light is absorbed into their surface, making them look yellowish and dull. If you want to whiten your teeth, the safest way is to focus on strengthening your teeth. People who strengthen soft teeth will notice they quickly begin to appear whiter as the enamel becomes smooth and hard. The more you strengthen your teeth, the more people will likely notice and comment on your white teeth, even without bleaching. Remember to check your teeth in natural lighting, since fluorescent lights (found in many bathrooms) will make teeth appear yellowish in color. Better than peering in a mirror, go outside and smile at a friend. Bleaching may temporarily help improve the color, but the process may damage or etch the surface, make it more porous, and ultimately make the tooth more sensitive and prone to staining. As you can see, bleaching teeth does not make them healthier and, if used, should be considered as a short-term whitening procedure that requires a longer follow-up therapy to repair tooth enamel luster and strength.

Negative Effects of Bleaching

In a laboratory study, human teeth were bleached and then tested for hardness. Results showed that bleaching decreased the hardness of the teeth, demineralizing and weakening them.[4] In 1991, before bleaching became big business, Dr. Harry Albers, the editor of a highly acclaimed dental newsletter, wrote an article stating that excessive whitening can break down tooth structure.[5]

Which products are safe, and which ones should you be careful about using? It is impossible to keep up with the evolving world of bleaching, but here is some basic, commonsense advice and guidance.

Many commercial products for whitening teeth carry dangers for you and for your teeth. Every dentist has seen side effects that include tooth sensitivity, damaged fillings, inflamed gums, something called *root resorption*—the disappearance of part of the root of your tooth—or a condition called *ankylosis*—the direct attachment of a tooth to the jawbone.[6]

I have never allowed my children or extended family to bleach their teeth. I bleached my teeth, only once, to try the new whitening strips. My teeth became sensitive, my gums became inflamed where they touched the strips, and any whitening was mild or undetectable.

In the past decade, bleaching has become a familiar treatment in many dental offices, and dentists sell kits for patients to use in their homes at night. You could easily be forgiven for assuming that with so many people using bleaching products, they must be well tested and safe. Interestingly, a survey showed that 92 percent of American dental schools teach their students night-guard bleaching techniques, sometimes instructed by salespeople from oral care companies.[7] The 8 percent of dental schools that do not participate cite lack of time as well as safety concerns. The facts are that in dental schools where bleaching is taught, students are told that only 25 percent of their patients will develop tooth sensitivity. Conservative reports indicate that following bleaching techniques, the number in reality is well over 50 percent.[8] The fact that some schools turn their back on bleaching and this disparity about sensitivity should tell you something.

I asked the ADA about controls on home-applied bleaching products, specifically bleaching mouth rinses. I wanted to know if the products had been tested and scrutinized in the same way that toothpastes were tested in the old days. I was told that some tests have been used for a few of the products, but only a limited number of companies conduct clinical trials today, citing expenses as prohibitive. The spokesperson told me it is impossible to control all the products in the marketplace, especially when there are so many new ones and when demand is so great. The public needs to know that there are only a few controls and that a lot of money changes hands. It would appear that, try as hard as it does, the ADA cannot protect you from all the bad products or the potential hazards on grocery store shelves. So learn for yourself what can happen, and know what to expect if things go wrong.

GUM RECESSION

Most whitening products contain peroxide as the main ingredient. Professionally applied bleaching products usually range from 10 percent (equivalent to 3 percent hydrogen peroxide) to 38 percent carbamide peroxide. Home-applied bleaching products are less concentrated but usually contain the same ingredients. In addition, many whitening toothpastes contain abrasive polishing agents to remove some of the surface layer of your tooth, the part most often stained. But remember, this layer offers your tooth the most protection from infection and a barrier to make teeth less sensitive.

The problem with hydrogen or carbamide peroxide is created by something called a *hydroxyl-free radical*, a by-product of bleaching that causes damage to the gums—damage that may be permanent.[9] If the bleaching agent touches your gums, it can irreversibly damage them, especially if it is strong. When dentists bleach teeth, they usually make a tray to prevent the bleaching agent from getting onto your gums or they protect your gums with a coating. Bleaching products could cause your gums to shrink back and expose a very sensitive part of your tooth. The gum damage may last for a few months or possibly for the rest of your life. This means that in reality you run the risk that your gums may never grow back. When gums recede, a space opens up between your teeth where your gums used to be. The new space looks like a black triangle between your teeth. You may even see the place where there is a join between the root and the crown of your tooth, the cementoenamel junction, which can easily become exposed. Not only will it look bad, it may cause you acute sensitivity too. A single bleaching treatment could cause this kind of damage. If you are going to bleach your teeth, you need to be very careful.

As I watch movies or TV or look at magazines, I am dismayed by the amount of gum recession I see on the teeth of celebrities and TV announcers. I hope they realize it is not just part of an aging process but a progressive, although preventable, problem. Take care if you bleach your teeth and remember that the big companies will tempt you to use their products with promises of glamorous white smiles.

The dentists who accept bleaching understand the risks and will always suggest minimizing tooth exposure to the lowest effective concentration: that is, by bleaching teeth for as little time as possible and with the weakest solution. The policy for pediatric dentists is that they should discourage "full-arch cosmetic bleaching for patients in the mixed dentition." (Mixed dentition is a stage that usually lasts well into the teenage years while all of the child's permanent teeth erupt.[10])

CANCER RISK

For decades, dentists and doctors have worried about the potential of hydrogen peroxide to cause cancer. I find it interesting that the people who originally sounded warning bells about whiteners— saying that they could cause or promote cancers[11]—have retracted these comments, stating they were premature.[12] An interesting case occurred in 1999 when the use of carbamide peroxide in a whitening agent called Opalescence was banned in the United Kingdom by the Department of Health and the Departments of Trade and Industry. The judgment was later overturned, and Opalescence became one of the most widely used dental office whitening products.[13] Other reports have linked the effects of bleaching to cellular changes seen in biological ionizing radiation, but these results were also later found to be "unsubstantiated."[14]

During the past two years the EPA has been studying whether there are differences in cancer risk between children and adults. Only since 2004 has there been any suggestion that children are at higher risk of cancer from childhood exposure than the same exposure during adulthood, and in some cases this has been shown to be a three-fold adjustment.[15] A review of the literature about bleaching would indicate that no one knows if peroxide exposure in children would be more harmful than in adults. Remember, any harmful effects of bleaching will be potentially increased by any increase in your risk factors: dry-mouth conditions, allergies, mouth infections, or acid reflux disease, for example.

With all the warnings officially overturned, I can tell you only that there are possible but unsubstantiated concerns about bleaching. I consider that a very well-known brand of whitening mouth rinse should be considered a co-carcinogen and that using the product may increase your risk for oral cancer. I do not suggest using any of these whitening products, but if you choose to use them, your only guide is that the ADA does not appear to give *harmful* whitening products their seal of acceptance.

People who smoke or who are at risk for cancer may want to take these *unsubstantiated* warnings very seriously. Stay clear of products that claim to whiten teeth, and realize that cancerous change often occurs slowly over time, with no immediate warning signal until it is too late.

My advice for people who continue to bleach their teeth is this: Choose only products that carry the ADA seal of acceptance. Use products for bleaching that have added fluoride to help recover lost tooth strength or finish up by using a fluoride rinse.

Bleaching Children's Teeth

The newly erupted front teeth of a seven- or eight-year-old child often appear as dull or yellow in color. The problem is caused partly because adult teeth are less white in contrast with baby teeth, but mainly because these newly erupted teeth always erupt with soft and porous enamel. New teeth take about a year to naturally mature as they absorb strengthening minerals onto their outside surface. When enamel is weak, there are watery spaces between the crystals that prevent light from reflecting off the surface. Light is absorbed by the softer enamel, which causes a soft tooth to look darker. The weaker the tooth, the darker it will look. Soft teeth also stain easily and are at risk for tooth decay and sensitivity. It makes far more sense to strengthen newly erupted teeth with xylitol and dilute fluoride mouth rinses than to potentially damage them internally or make them weaker with bleaching. Softened enamel has pores that absorb color from foods and drinks and can turn a tooth a dull brown or gray.

Teeth may have an unattractive color for a couple of other reasons, including some "good stains." Good stains are seen on teeth when dental disease has been rapidly controlled, when the remnants of thick plaque and harmful bacteria die off quickly. The debris collects around the tooth, often looking like a dark stain at the gum line. Patients may be concerned at first, whereas in reality this stain is the sign of improved oral health, less bleeding, and a healthier mouth and gums. A dental cleaning will quickly remove this kind of staining and leave the healthier teeth pristine and white.

Sometimes colors are embedded in teeth; such stains are usually caused by taking medications or from infection that became built into a tooth while it was forming. These deep or intrinsic stains are very hard to improve or remove and even professional bleaching may do little to help. Often, placing veneers or artificial covers on the outside of the tooth is the only way to mask this kind of staining.

Teeth thickness increases with age, much as a tree increases its girth as the years go by. Teeth do not increase in their overall size, but the inner dentin layer keeps growing thicker over the years, gradually reducing the size of the pulp in the center of the tooth, until it may completely disappear in a very old tooth. For this reason, in a young tooth there is a shorter distance from the outside to the live part in the center. The tubes that run through the dentin are also wider in a young tooth, because dentin is also deposited inside them until, in elderly teeth, the tube holes may be completely blocked. For these reasons, bleach can run along the wide-open tubes of a young tooth and will probably do more damage to the living part in the center of the tooth than to an older tooth. When you bleach a tooth, the live cells inside can easily become irritated during treatment.

An overview of side effects, benefits, and concerns about bleaching teeth was covered in a report from 2003.[16] Studies concluded that bleaching inflames the living tissue (pulp) in the center of the tooth, and in an adult tooth, the changes take between two and eight weeks to disappear. In some cases the living pulp can die. I advise you to be cautious about allowing young children or teenagers to bleach their teeth with any regularity, at least until more independent, unbiased studies are available.

Does Bleaching Last?

Results from patient interviews and sponsored research indicate that the color of almost all teeth can be whitened and that improvements can be maintained for a number of years.[17] Bleaching removes surface stains, but at the same time, this treatment may increase the porosity of a tooth. Hydrogen peroxide is released from the bleaching product and travels through the spaces to the deeper layers inside the tooth, even into the sensitive dentin. Studies done on dogs in the 1980s indicated that when peroxide enters the pulp chamber of teeth during bleaching, the stronger the solution, the more peroxide enters the center of the tooth. Some studies showed hemorrhaging and inflammation in the pulp, although it reversed over time.[18] Later studies showed changes in the special odontoblast cells, and since these are the cells that form new dentin throughout the life of a tooth, this could potentially be a very serious complication for a young tooth.[19]

For an adult with badly stained teeth, bleaching may seem to be a starting point from which to begin new dental care routines. My suggestion would be to work for several months to strengthen teeth before bleaching them. If improvements are noticeable, you may want to consider one or two years of strengthening teeth before attempting to bleach them. At the very least, use strengthening treatments to protect your enamel from damage both before and immediately after any bleaching treatments. Repeated bleaching of a tooth may make it look whiter, but it can also make teeth look dull and lifeless, because the enamel layer has been made porous, so it no longer reflects light in a healthy way, rather like overly dyed hair that loses its shine.

One young man I know had whitened his teeth with unsafe products to the point where they were about to crumble and break at the gum level. His teeth were the color of opaque paper. One day he accidentally hit his tooth against a coffee cup, and a small piece chipped off. This was the moment he began regular use of the system I recommend, and within two years he was able to restore his teeth to health. Now, five years later, his teeth gleam white again, brighter than ever and with the shine of dental health, and no bleaching treatments. Last winter he slipped and fell, hitting *all* his front teeth against a hard metal rail. He was very anxious to assess what damage had been done and was happy to find that his teeth were so strong, no damage had occurred.

Bleaching and Fillings

There are special concerns about bleaching for people who have silver fillings in their teeth. The peroxide in bleaching agents has been shown to affect silver fillings, possibly releasing mercury from them. I recently read a study about drain cleaners used to clean the plumbing lines in dental offices. I was intrigued to read that little pieces of filling in the drain gave off mercury vapor when they interacted with various cleaners. In the study, pieces of silver filling were treated with various drain-cleaning chemicals, including chlorine, ammonia, and hydrogen peroxide. It appeared that a 7 percent solution of hydrogen peroxide released the most mercury from the silver amalgam filling material, more than 400 times more mercury than the control (plain water). I later found studies from the early 1990s showing that mercury from silver fillings goes into the solution following exposure to peroxide in bleaching agents.[20] This information is a great health concern not only for people who bleach their teeth but also for anyone using hydrogen peroxide as a mouth rinse.

People with white fillings also face a danger from bleaching teeth if they have leaky fillings or any teeth that have early decay or unfilled cavities. Any bleaching liquid that seeps directly into the unprotected tooth is likely to kill the nerve of the tooth. You must also be aware that a filling or a crown will not bleach. If you want to avoid a zebra-like appearance, you need to make sure which teeth have fillings in them before you start.

Bleaching with Laser

Most recently, the U.S. Food and Drug Administration (FDA) approved bleaching with laser for use in dental offices. These special lights bleach an entire mouth of teeth in about two minutes, and the effect is supposed to last for a couple of years. Because the equipment deals with one tooth at a time, it is said to help people with varying colored teeth even out the colors. Laser bleaching apparently is less stressful for the nerve inside a tooth, which suggests there is less chance of killing a tooth with this method.

Questions to Ask Before Bleaching

In summary, think carefully before using an off-the-shelf bleach system. Ask yourself who is looking out for the health of your teeth—oral care companies or you? Don't leave your dental health to others; learn about the risks of tooth whitening and evaluate the potential problems. Most bleaching agents sensitize and soften your teeth and, used improperly, can cause gum recession or tooth weakening. If you are going to bleach your teeth, you need to understand that the idea of tooth whitening may sound better than it really is, and that by building strength into your teeth you will naturally and safely lighten and brighten them, no matter your age or the color of your teeth when you start.

PART FIVE

The Good News

The patient's best interest, above all other considerations, is paramount.

—Elliott Moskowitz, editor, *New York State Dental Journal*, Spring 2006

CHAPTER ELEVEN

Food for Teeth

Most people today are aware that ingredients in food can have either positive or negative effects on health. As a teenager in England, I started to eat a diet of unrefined foods and products that were as natural as possible. I chose whole-grain cereal, live-culture yogurt, nuts, and other foods I hoped would promote good health. Such products were never seen on grocery shelves, but they were available from special health food stores. At that time, people ridiculed these unusual diets and generally referred to people like me as health food nuts.

Achieving Balance

It has always seemed logical to me that a natural and unrefined diet would be better for health, and I am prepared to imagine that a carefully balanced diet may prevent and even reverse certain medical conditions. I found that my health food diet of whole grains, vitamins, and lots of fresh vegetables drastically reduced my teenage acne, which was enough to make me a believer. I use the word *believer* because there seems to be no way to know with scientific certainty if organic health foods really are better than the ordinary ones from grocery stores. Our family has always chosen to avoid artificial ingredients and limit sugar to the minimum needed for taste.

Today the idea of whole grains, vitamins, and natural products has become big business. Every mainstream grocery store carries a range of unrefined products, and now it is accepted, even fashionable, to buy foods that are organic and free of pesticides and chemicals.

Even though information surfaces constantly about the health benefits of special foods, plenty of confusion and misinformation for consumers remains. Many people are so afraid of the words "salt," "fat," and "sugar" that they search frantically to find items that are free of these ingredients. Strangely, people are prepared to substitute artificial chemicals about which they know nothing simply to avoid their natural equivalents. Recently I talked with a new mother who gave up sugar during pregnancy and replaced all sugar-containing items with diet ones. Her pregnancy did not go well, and she wonders if she would have been healthier cutting back on sugar instead of using chemical sweeteners in its place.

Sugar Substitutes

Many people understand the difference between natural and artificial ingredients, yet few realize that there is a similar dichotomy in the world of sugar substitutes. Most people imagine that sugar replacements are all artificial products, but this is not true. A number of natural sugarless sweeteners are derived from plants, although most people are familiar only with the artificial ones. For instance, sweeteners like stevia and xylitol are derived from natural sources and are healthy and safe sugar substitutes, despite the fact that they have such off-putting and chemical-sounding names. Artificial sweeteners, on the other hand, often have alluring names like Splenda, Sweet'N Low, and Equal. Artificial sweeteners have been promoted in the United States for decades, giving consumers confidence to assume they are safe, but in the world of sweeteners, names and appearances can be deceptive.

Reading the labels on foods is important for the sake of our health, and dental health is no exception, since the sugarless world is equally confusing. There are great differences for teeth between the effects of consuming the natural and dentally beneficial sugar substitute xylitol and xylitol's ugly stepsister, the artificial sugarless sweetener called *sorbitol.*

XYLITOL VERSUS SORBITOL

Breath mints often contain ordinary sugar or sorbitol. Sugar feeds bad-breath bacteria, giving them extra energy to produce acids that can destroy teeth, but although sorbitol is a good-tasting artificial sugar substitute, it may generate thicker plaque and in this way be dentally unsafe for teeth. Recently a chewing gum containing xylitol has been heavily promoted in the U.S. marketplace, even in dental offices. It appears that the gum contains xylitol for oral health, because the wrapper advertises "now with xylitol!" The statement is confusing, even misleading, because the main ingredient in this sugar-free gum is sorbitol and other artificial sweeteners, combined with only a small amount of xylitol. The amount of xylitol in each piece is so small it would be difficult to consume enough each day to enjoy the dental benefits that xylitol offers without experiencing the negative effects from sorbitol and the other artificial sweeteners.

Sorbitol is an artificial, laboratory-produced sweetener that has FDA safety clearance to replace sugar in candies, drinks, and confectionaries, but the product can cause gastric problems like bloating and stomach cramps at low dosage and should never be given to children under three. Possibly the biggest problem with sorbitol is that plaque bacteria on teeth learn to use it as an energy source in order to grow and thicken. Many people who consume sorbitol find they develop acid reflux symptoms which themselves can be damaging to teeth. Sorbitol is cheap, so it is often mixed together with more expensive sweeteners like xylitol. It takes chewing about three sticks of sorbitol-containing gum for harmful bacteria to modify themselves and learn to use the sweetener. Studies show that when bacteria have energy from sorbitol, they sustain themselves, grow, and multiply,[1] which may cause gum irritation or gum disease. If your teenager is experiencing gum disease, cavities, or acid reflux, consider eliminating sorbitol-containing drinks, candy, and gum. Dental, gastric, and even acid reflux problems often improve when products containing 100 percent xylitol are used instead of those made with sorbitol.

For many years the only alternative ingredient for sugar in popular gum and candy was sorbitol.[2] Finally, the United States marketplace is starting to enjoy the option of alternative and natural sugar substitutes in candies, mints, and chewing gum. Xylitol is a sugarless and healthy choice that is dentally safe for teeth and has additional benefits to clean and strengthen teeth with continuous use.[3]

CAN SUGAR-FREE FOODS CAUSE DAMAGE?

Often at my seminars I notice people in the audience sipping fruited diet drinks or snacking on sugar-free mints and chewing gum. As people learn more about preventing cavities and gum disease, they are shocked to discover how these diet, sugar-free products can contribute to cavities and even promote harmful mouth bacteria.

Decoding product labels is a time-consuming problem. It may be difficult to decide if sugar-free or diet items are safe for teeth and figure out which ones are beneficial and which less healthful. Don't believe that when a product says it is sugar free it means it is "safe or good for teeth." As we have just discussed, sugar-free products, especially chewing gum and diet drinks, may contain sorbitol. Another problem is that many diet drinks that contain no sugar will attack your teeth because they are viciously acidic. Diet soda, for example, is sugar free, yet it will cause as much—and possibly more—dental damage than a sugar-containing drink.[4]

Even children's sugarless chewable vitamins can contain a dentally harmful, non-digestible substance called *oligosaccharide*, which is regarded as sugar free because it has no calories. But oligosaccharides are not safe for teeth since they give energy to harmful bacteria and in this way can potentially cause cavities.[5]

Health professionals in every field—especially those involved in prenatal care—are important sources of information for parents. School administrators likewise play a big part in improving the overall health and dental health of children in the United States. In Scandinavia, community health programs include dietary advice at individual and group levels. That advice focuses on avoiding acidic beverages and eating tooth-protective foods at the end of each meal. In Switzerland, the use of safe-for-teeth candies and confectionaries is encouraged in schools. Perhaps looking at the subject of nutrition from a more global perspective could help Americans escape the controls of food lobbies and special-interest agendas.

Today 30 percent of carbonated beverages in the United States are sweetened with the artificial sweetener aspartame. Alitame, aspartame, saccharin, and sucralose are sweeteners synthesized in laboratories. (For anyone interested in learning more about the world of sweeteners, Dr. Joseph Mercola and Dr. Kendra Degen Pearsall have published a comprehensive book called *Sweet Deception*, which reviews the dangers of artificial sweeteners and food additives and provides interesting information on this subject.[6])

As we have seen, sugar-free sweeteners like sorbitol can actually cause bacteria in your mouth to change and thicken.[7] Remember, by your third stick of gum, mouth bacteria may adapt to sorbitol and begin to use it as an energy source.[8] A recent study compared plaque and mouth bacteria in two groups eating sugar-free gum. One group chewed xylitol gum and the other chewed gum sweetened with sorbitol and maltitol. The number of harmful mouth bacteria went down in the xylitol group, but there was no change in the sorbitol group.[9] If you routinely alternate sugar with sorbitol or if you eat sorbitol-containing products and have bad breath or gum disease, try to eliminate sorbitol from your diet and replace it with products sweetened with 100 percent xylitol.

Nutritional guidelines can be confusing, and they seem to change at an alarming speed. We once learned about the evils of eating chocolate and then discovered that *good* chocolate contains an ingredient with health and dental benefits. For a long time salt was considered bad, but as with chocolate, evidence now shows that *good* salt contains minerals that may actually improve health.[10]

It is sometimes hard for a consumer to separate fact from fiction. Besides the difficulty of identifying a truly healthful food, how can we be certain about the effect it is having on our bodies? A manufacturer may claim that some product is good for you, but how do you know if it is true? There are just so many variables. Fear tactics and poor research confuse the public and help manufacturers reap profits at the expense of our health. Fortunately, in the case of teeth, results can be easily monitored. You could use your next dental checkup to determine if replacing sorbitol with 100 percent xylitol products has created a positive impact on your oral health.

Which Water Is Best?

Part of my dental detective work was to find foods and drinks that would protect teeth. By ending a meal with something nonacidic, teeth would be saved from the damage of sugary or acidic items or drinks consumed during the meal. My first search was for drinks that might protect teeth. Unfortunately, few alkaline drinks are available, and even tap water may be acidic. A few mineral waters are alkaline and could be used to protect teeth after eating something acidic. To learn more about the acidity/alkalinity measurement, or pH, of water, you can measure it with special litmus paper or check to see whether the pH of bottled water is listed on its label. (I describe pH measurement in greater detail in chapter 5.) On the Internet, www.mineralwaters.org can give information about mineral waters and has a list of their pH.[11] As a generalization, the more expensive bottled waters, originating from various regions of the world, seem to be alkaline. The pH of cheaper and more commonly available bottled waters, however, is usually acidic, sometimes because of additives in them. Evian is a brand of bottled water that is mildly alkaline, with a pH of 7.2, and Fiji water, from the island of Fiji, has a pH of 7.4.

If you are at risk for cavities and drink a lot of tap water, it may be important to check the pH of this water regularly because it appears to vary as a result of, possibly, additives to public water supplies.[12] People who wake and need a drink during the night, people with a dry mouth, or those who are dehydrated or sick may want to take particular interest in the pH value of the water they are consuming.

Well water and city water may have different pH levels from season to season and from month to month, and testing them is the only way to determine their pH. The water supply to my home in Rochester usually tests acidic, for instance, whereas in San Antonio, it tests alkaline.

Citric Acid

Citric acid is damaging in any mouth, and in a dry mouth, where it is not diluted or washed off teeth by saliva, the damage will be more extreme. Citric acid can initiate a chain of events that concludes with calcium being pulled out of tooth enamel and either swallowed or deposited into infected plaque on teeth. Here is a simplified version of the events: Citric acid chelates, or clumps, the calcium in your saliva—in much the same way that lemon juice added to milk makes the milk curdle or clump together—and you swallow it. When the calcium is gone from your saliva, a chemical suction is created, and calcium is pulled out from your teeth to fill this void. Minerals dissolve from teeth, weakening them and making the enamel thinner, softer, and more sensitive.

I once consulted with a man who was suffering from numerous dental problems including rapid buildup of hardened plaque and a substance often referred to as tartar on his teeth. He described scraping these deposits off his teeth daily to try to control the problem. We talked about the things he ate and drank, searching for a source of acidity in his diet. He had no acid reflux, took no medications, and indulged in no unusual food habits. He did drink a lot of water because he lived in a desert area and his mouth was often dry. He had tested his tap water and found it was neutral, at pH 7.0. I was convinced his problem was caused by acidity, and we continued to talk until we discovered that to mask the chlorine taste in his tap water, he added citric acid—the juice of a lemon—to it.

The tart taste of citric acid is very refreshing. Many fruits contain citric acid, as do the drinks made from them: grapefruit, oranges, limes, or lemons. Many sports and health drinks also contain citric acid, which quenches the thirst of someone who is dehydrated after exercise or is parched on a hot summer day. Citric acid is often selected by people with chronic dry mouth—athletes, those on mouth-drying medications, and the sick or debilitated. Lemon juice, high in citric acid, is unfortunately often chosen in nursing homes to swab or clean the teeth of elderly patients unable to brush their teeth themselves.

In another case, a twenty-year-old came to consult with me about three root-canal treatments she had just completed and the crowns she was working so hard to pay for. She had spent an enormous amount of money on dental repairs, and still her teeth were miserably sensitive, especially to cold. She told me she could no longer eat ice cream or enjoy chilled drinks, and that the problem seemed to be getting worse. Her dentist had told her she was simply unlucky: she had thin enamel and soft teeth.

I never accept an excuse of soft teeth; I will always search for reasons that explain why someone has dental problems. I asked what kinds of foods and drinks she consumed most often. We tested the pH of her bottled water and found it to be neutral, so it was not the problem. We discussed acid reflux and other reasons for mouth acidity. We talked about her diet, and not until we went through her daily foods, starting with breakfast, did we discover the reason for her damaged enamel. This young lady was of Turkish background, and her family tradition was to suck a lemon wedge before and after eating. Bingo! She habitually sucked lemons against her teeth after every meal and snack. In fact, she ate a quantity of citrus fruits throughout the day, never considering that healthy fruits could be causing her dental damage.

My suggestion to both the man with plaque buildup and the young Turkish woman was either to change their habit of using lemons or to protect their teeth after every acidic episode with some kind of tooth-friendly food, preferably xylitol. (The next chapter describes this product and its benefits in great detail.) If xylitol is not available, other foods, such as bananas, almonds, potatoes, vegetables of all kinds, fresh apples, and even pineapple, can make the mouth alkaline. If you have a favorite habit or snack, you may want to make sure your frequent treat is not damaging your teeth.

Diet and Energy Drinks

Diet drinks can be as acidic as drinks with sugar in them, and it often surprises people to discover that fresh pure fruit juices can be damaging to teeth. Parents should note that although fresh apples will clean teeth and make the mouth alkaline, apple juice is strongly acidic, and even diluted, it has the potential of being extremely damaging to a baby's or a toddler's teeth. Teeth should be protected with xylitol or some other tooth-protective food after drinking it.

While diet drinks do not have any sugar in them, they are usually acidic and therefore very damaging to teeth. Gatorade and energy drinks like Red Bull each have a pH value around 3.2. Most carbonated sodas, like Coke and Pepsi, contain phosphoric acids that create an acidity level typically around pH 2.8 (go to www.cleanwhiteteeth.com for a list of beverage pH levels). Think about the acidity of sodas or other drinks you may enjoy, especially if you have dental problems or believe you have "weak teeth." The best news is that the problem can be solved without having to give up your favorite food or drink. Just use xylitol or other tooth-protective food to take the acidity from your mouth.

Most energy drinks also contain a mixture of sugars and syrups. Glucose sugar is used to increase the energy content of a drink without changing the taste or smell of the product and therefore it is often an ingredient in health or athletic drinks. Studies show that harmful bacteria in the mouth gain substantial energy from glucose, which increases the likelihood of tooth decay and damage, especially in a dry mouth.

Protection with Xylitol

Elderly or special-needs patients, especially those on mouth-drying medications, may be given booster drinks as meal replacements. These drinks often contain glucose, citric acids, and other tooth-softening ingredients. Cleaning the mouth with xylitol or even adding it to the drink may help control dental disease for these patients. Glucose is also used in shakes and food-drinks for children and toddlers, and these drinks can precipitate especially bad dental problems, especially for anyone with a dry mouth. The exciting fact is that protecting teeth can be as simple as ending the meal with a xylitol breath mint, candy, or chewing gum or by using a xylitol mouth spray.

Glucose syrups are also found as ingredients in powdered infant formulas, including soy formula. Because of this, formulas are usually not safe for a baby's teeth. After feeding a soy formula product to a baby, wipe any erupted teeth with the xylitol solution described in the next chapter. Xylitol-containing tooth wipes called Spiffies are convenient to use and are available on the Internet at www.spiffies. com.[13] Spiffies were developed by Dr. Ray Wagner, a pediatrician who became concerned about this problem after providing emergency care for a child with grossly decayed baby teeth.

Adult wipes with a length of floss attached to one side, called Floss and Wipe, are also available. Using xylitol to adjust the acidity of your mouth gives you an easy and natural way to protect your teeth from potential harm.

Cariostatic Food

Several foods are not only safe for teeth but also have tooth-protective or anti-cavity features. Some of them are so effective they are called *cariostatic* because they stop cavities from forming. These foods may also contain minerals to boost the strength of teeth, or they may form a coating over teeth that can protect enamel from the cavity-forming process.

COW'S MILK

One of the most cariostatic foods for teeth is cow's milk. Many people are concerned about milk because they know it contains a sugar called *lactose*. Bacteria in the mouth can break down lactose to form lactic acid, but the acidity level of lactic acid (its pH) is not low enough to dissolve teeth. In fact, milk contains so many helpful, cavity-stopping properties that it is not only safe for but also protective of teeth. Experiments in 1984 showed that if you drink milk while eating something acidic or sweet that would otherwise damage your teeth,[14] the calcium and phosphate in it will prevent enamel damage.[15] Perhaps this fact is the rationale for eating cookies with a glass of milk! Here's an added tip: If someone's tooth is knocked out by accident and he or she is able to take it to a dentist for implantation, carry it in a container of saliva, saline solution, or milk.

CHEESE AND CHOCOLATE

Cheese has similar cavity-preventing qualities. Cheese raises the alkalinity of the mouth and increases the amount of calcium around teeth, which helps rebuild damaged enamel. The protective effects of cheese are seen even when cheese is baked. Experiments conducted in the late 1990s showed that eating cheese after meals and as a snack can be very protective, especially for young children.[16] In one experiment, seven- to nine-year-old children ate a small piece of cheese after breakfast for two years. At the end of the controlled study, researchers found significantly less tooth damage in these children when compared to a similar group that did not eat cheese after breakfast.[17]

For mothers who have problems weaning their children from juice-filled sippy cups, putting half a teaspoon of xylitol into water as a replacement may work, but if not, frequent snacks of cubed cheese or yogurt can help compensate for damage done by the juice drinks.

And for adults who find their favorite wine to be acidic, now you have a good reason to enjoy a cube of cheese as an accompanying snack!

The addition of certain foods at mealtimes, especially dairy products, can provide a balance to protect teeth from the dangers of any potentially harmful ingredients contained in the meal. In England as I grew up most meals were completed with a piece of cheese. Note that people with food allergies, particularly those who are lactose intolerant and therefore cannot derive any protection from dairy products, may need extra help to prevent dental problems.

A 1940s sugar study showed that even chocolate has a protective effect, making sugar less harmful to teeth.[18] People who were extremely vulnerable to tooth decay were given dark chocolate to eat between meals, while others were given plain sugar. Those who ate dark chocolate had fewer cavities than those who ate comparable amounts of regular sugar. Something in chocolate exerted a protective effect on teeth. In 1986, a cocoa factor extracted from chocolate was shown to have cavity-preventing abilities.[19] Milk chocolate contains so little of this cocoa factor, though, that its other ingredients may override these protective effects.

PLANT FIBERS AND LEAVES

Similar protective and cariostatic factors have been found in certain plant fibers and leaves. Dental professionals have been intrigued that people who regularly chew sugarcane have little tooth decay. The protection appears to come from a substance in the fibers called *phytate*,[20] which sticks to the tooth surface and forms a coating that protects tooth enamel from damage.

Some foods, such as fresh apples and tea, contain *polyphenols* that control mouth bacteria and thus have a protective effect on teeth.[21] Trigonelline is the ingredient in coffee responsible for its aroma and taste, and it also has antibacterial properties. According to a 2005 study at the University of Ancona in Italy, coffee may cause mouth bacteria to be less adhesive and therefore less able to stick to teeth.[22]

INTENSE SWEETENERS

Some sweeteners that are natural and healthy are nevertheless *several thousand times* sweeter than sugar, which is why they are called *intense sweeteners*. Their names are often difficult to pronounce: glyrrihizin comes from licorice root, and thaumatin and mirakulin occur in fruits. New research shows that licorice may eliminate harmful mouth bacteria, although many of the systems involved are not fully understood. Dr. Wenyuan Shi and Dr. Max Anderson, of the Department of Oral Biology in the School of Dentistry at the University of California–Los Angeles, identified a specific herbal formula extracted from Chinese licorice root that targets and disables the bacteria of dental disease. Dr. Shi has worked to develop a lollipop that contains this licorice product mixed with other cariostatic plant extracts.

Similarly, a study of cranberry juice at the University of Rochester showed that it contains components that protect teeth.[23] Commercially bottled cranberry juice, unfortunately, is usually a cocktail of sugar and many other juices that are often very harmful to teeth.

PROPOLIS

Other studies have shown the tooth-protection properties of propolis, a sticky substance made by honeybees to protect their hives.[24] Propolis has been used for thousands of years as an antimicrobial in folk medicine. Propolis appears to inhibit a key enzyme that is necessary for the formation of dental plaque, and the amount of protection varies with the concentration of propolis. Years ago, a retired dentist told me how he successfully used raw honey to heal infected gums, before the advent of gum treatments and periodontal specialists. At that time, his dental colleagues ridiculed him for the idea, believing that he was putting sugar into people's mouths. Perhaps today, his treatments would be admired.

Honey itself may have health and dental benefits, but study results are conflicting, with some even suggesting that it may in fact cause cavities.[25] Gluconic and other acids are present in honey, and its pH can vary between pH 3.9 and 6.1.[26] Processed honey is very different from raw honey; it often contains added sugar, has a low pH, and in this way may contribute to dental problems. Coconut milk is another low pH food that should be viewed as a potential cause of tooth decay when left on teeth for extended periods of time.

For many years dentists have known that finishing a meal or a snack with something dentally healthy can alter the chemistry of your mouth and leave it safe for teeth. At mealtimes fifty years ago children and adults would usually accompany and complete their meals with water, milk, or tea. Today the majority of people in the United States drink acidic drinks before and after meals: sodas, flavored waters, or sparkling juices. Changing the drink you consume with meals or at least the last thing on your teeth at the end of a meal may be enough to help you avoid fillings and cavities.

The most important thing is to know at least one or two foods that you like and which are safe for teeth so that you can eat these to complete any meal or snack made up of foods that are damaging. The best part about my system for dental health is that it does not require you to give up your favorite food or drink, no matter how damaging it may appear. All you need is to understand which products are dangerous for teeth and the things that put you at risk for tooth damage. Armed with this knowledge, you can use tooth-friendly, protective foods to win the war against cavities and enjoy a life of controlled and improved dental health.

CHAPTER TWELVE

Xylitol

Xylitol (pronounced ZIE-lih-tol) was originally used a hundred years ago as an intravenous support for diabetic patients who had to undergo surgery. Xylitol was used because of its safety, its freedom from the insulin pathway, and its ability to keep patients stable during surgical procedures. It was originally extracted from the woody fibers of birch trees, although today xylitol comes from such other sources as vegetables, fruits, corn husks, and a variety of other hardwoods. In its granular form xylitol looks and tastes like ordinary table sugar, but with a slightly fruity overtone. The difference, however, is that xylitol is not only tooth friendly but also has amazing benefits for teeth and general health.

Xylitol can be used as one of the most effective methods for removing harmful cavity-forming bacteria from the mouth. Eating a little less than two teaspoons (6.5 grams) of xylitol daily will gradually eliminate the harmful germs that normally feed on sugar or carbohydrates to produce mouth acidity, cause cavities and promote ear, nose and throat infections. It takes five weeks to eradicate the harmful bacteria from plaque on teeth and about six months to clean the tongue, saliva, throat, and other areas of the mouth of these bacteria.

The Early History of Xylitol

The idea of using wood sugar to protect teeth is old, despite the fact that it is a new concept in the United States. Since ancient times, people have cleaned their teeth with instruments made from wood. In parts of Africa, intricately carved dental sticks are highly prized and stored in special wooden boxes. Native Americans were known to bite into birch wood and chew wooden sticks cut from birch trees as a cure for bad breath, and they gave their babies teething rattles carved from birch wood. They also seemed to be aware of the antifungal and antibacterial effects of birch wood, and they stored precious medicines and herbs inside wraps of birch-tree bark. Young Turkish children chew a raw gum from birch trees, and in rural areas of Northern Europe and Russia today, children are encouraged as their teeth erupt to drink the juice from birch trees.

In a country where birch forests are plentiful, it is not surprising that during the 1940s, the Finnish Sugar Company became the first company to extract and distribute xylitol commercially. When there was a shortage of regular sugar during World War II, xylitol was used in the kitchens and on the tables of Europe. Now, sixty years later, more than half the candy produced in Scandinavia is made with xylitol, and the Scandinavians have regular dental health programs in elementary schools and kindergarten where children are provided with it. In Finland, xylitol chewing gum sales have increased from 1 percent in 1977 to 54 percent in 1998.[1] Switzerland has a variety of tooth-friendly candy made from xylitol, and travelers to Asia will find candy counters everywhere filled with gum and mints sweetened with xylitol.

Xylitol first arrived in the United States as an ingredient in chewing gum in the 1970s, but there was little interest in health food or natural cures at that time. The first xylitol gum tasted somewhat bland and was flavored with licorice, being rated a poor competitor to the tastier gum that the American marketplace normally enjoyed. Today xylitol can be purchased in granular form as well as in tooth-friendly zellies, breath mints and gum, tooth gels, mouth rinses, baby products, and nasal sprays. Products are in most health food stores, vitamin outlets, and even some of the more progressive grocery stores that feature organic and natural products.

Recent Studies

During large, long-term dental studies from 1989 to 1994 undertaken in Belize, Central America, researchers noticed at the start of the program that some people's teeth showed signs of early cavities. These teeth were reevaluated at the end of the studies, and researchers documented that the decay had stabilized in the xylitol group in both the outer tooth enamel and inner dentin, and in some of the cases, the decay had completely healed.[2]

More recently, the Finnish Dr. Pentti Alanen completed a six-year study that examined the effectiveness of various xylitol products in preventing cavities. He showed that a daily dose of 5 grams of xylitol, either in mints or gum, had preventive effects among the 740 children, ages ten to twelve, who participated in the study. After two years, there was an approximately 50 percent reduction in decay in the xylitol groups compared with the control groups, with no other difference in dental care. The study also showed that if xylitol was used regularly for a sufficient period, a three-month break in the regimen did not reduce its effect.[3]

Other studies have demonstrated how well xylitol works in all age groups. In 2006, for example, Dr. Peter Milgrom of the University of Washington presented a study that shows exactly how much xylitol must be eaten each day to create a reduction in the harmful bacteria around teeth. He found that a dose of 6.5 grams each day for five weeks reduced the bacteria in plaque on teeth and that after six months the bacteria were gone from the saliva and skin of the mouth and tongue. He also showed that when the dosage is continued for two years, less plaque forms, and the effects can be long-lived.[4]

Lower doses may offer teeth immediate protection from mouth acidity, but research shows that consuming less than 6 grams daily may not give positive bacteria changes. Higher doses may have some general health benefits, but from a dental point of view, teeth benefit from 6.5 to 10 grams of xylitol each day, after which the effects plateau, or level off. Eating more than 10 grams a day will not reduce mouth bacteria any faster, nor reduce the time it takes to effect the change. More research may reveal other features of dosage, but for now people are encouraged to make a regular routine of eating a little xylitol after every meal and snack.

Higher doses of xylitol have been suggested for women who suffer osteoporosis. It appears that xylitol has a benefit on the absorption of calcium into the body and for this reason, it helps in the repair and mineralization of the skeleton. Doctors who believe in alkalizing the body for health often suggest around 20 grams of xylitol each day for alkalizing benefits that are believed to promote improved health. Some doctors even believe that there is a group of eight special sugars, from among the more than eight hundred known sugars, that are essential for health. Xylose—the precursor of xylitol—is one of these specific sugars, and doctors believe that these sugars provide the building blocks that enable cells in your body to communicate effectively and understand which cells are good and which ones are bad. These eight special sugars are sold in a supplement form.

Harmful bacteria are unable to use xylitol as an energy source, and as they become starved, their numbers on and around teeth gradually reduce. Bacteria absorb xylitol as they do regular sugar, but any attempt to process it is unsuccessful. The bacteria continue trying, but they use up their resources in this futile effort. As the bacteria die out, new ones take their place that are less adhesive than the original ones and more easily removed from teeth by brushing and rinsing. After eating xylitol regularly for two years, most people notice that plaque no longer accumulates in any quantity around teeth. An important fact to know is that studies show harmful mouth bacteria (mutans streptococci) do not adapt to xylitol, even after years of exposure to it.[5]

The Many Benefits of Eating Xylitol

As studies have shown, eating a little xylitol can rebuild and strengthen teeth over time and may completely prevent the need for a filling for an impending cavity. Xylitol stimulates a natural healing process in teeth, and eating some xylitol makes teeth feel smoother while helping to keep them cleaner. If you are among the millions of people who suffer from sensitive teeth, cavities, or plaque buildup, xylitol may help to alleviate some of these problems as well.

Research further shows that xylitol can reduce plaque formation and cavities; it makes sense, then, to think that it may simultaneously reduce other infections connected with the nose, mouth, throat, and possibly the lungs. Future studies will improve our understanding about changes in mouth chemistry and biology and possibly confirm if measures like eating a little xylitol each day could help people of all ages, particularly the disabled and debilitated, enjoy improved general health.[6] It certainly seems possible that studies of the future may hold harmful mouth bacteria responsible for some of the more complicated medical problems that debilitated and disabled people suffer.

XYLITOL AND EAR INFECTIONS

If you think about the connection between tooth bacteria and ear infections for a few minutes, you will understand that the mouth or oral cavity is connected to the throat, the nose and nasal passages, the sinuses, and the tubes that go from the back of your throat and into your ears. Xylitol has the effect of reducing the number of sticky plaque bacteria on teeth, and it appears that it may reduce the number of sticky bacteria responsible for ear infections in the tubes that travel from the throat into the ears. As harmful bacteria disappear, xylitol-tolerant non-sticky bacteria take their place. More research with xylitol appears each year, and eating a little xylitol daily may be an avenue to consider for any child suffering ear infections, sinus problems, or allergies.

In Finland during the 1950s, doctors were intrigued by the fact that the number of ear infections for preschool children decreased as the numbers of harmful bacteria around teeth was reduced. Since then a number of studies have shown that young children experienced around 42 percent fewer ear infections, known as *otitis media*, when they ate xylitol regularly.[7]

In 2000 the American Academy of Pediatrics reported that doctors wrote more than 800 prescriptions for every 1,000 children they treated for ear infections. This is of special concern since frequent use of antibiotics can develop drug-resistant bacteria strains. Children with recurrent ear infections are at higher risk for learning problems, not to mention the pain and suffering these children and their families experience. Clinical trials show that chewing xylitol gum, candies, or mints sweetened with 100 percent xylitol five times a day may reduce ear infection without antibiotics. Xylitol-based nasal sprays are also available and may be useful to treat sinusitis and allergies.[8]

XYLITOL AND CAVITY PREVENTION

Adults who regularly eat around two teaspoons of xylitol (in any form) each day can remove 95 percent of cavity-forming germs from their mouths within six months. Anyone who continues to eat xylitol will notice less plaque forming on their teeth, and the need for dental cleanings will gradually be reduced or eliminated. New parents can use the xylitol mouth-cleaning system in the most exciting way of all—to help control the transmission of harmful bacteria to their babies and limit the chance of their children having a cavity by 70 to 90 percent.[9]

Xylitol not only reduces harmful mouth bacteria but also works to raise the pH in the mouth and to stimulate a healthy flow of saliva. In this way it helps protect your teeth. Since 1970 there have been hundreds of studies to show xylitol's ability to limit, decrease, and even repair cavities. While xylitol exerts its powerful effect on cavity-forming bacteria, it also shows the ability to stimulate the repair of soft spots on teeth, often seen as the first stage of a cavity forming.[10] A recent study with special-needs children shows clearly how xylitol can strengthen and heal teeth.[11]

Although it may seem ironic, this sweet and delicious xylose derivative could be the ultimate magic bullet for tooth decay, working with nature to change the chemistry and biology of a dentally dangerous mouth to bring it back to health in less than a year.

Strong, healthy teeth need to be bathed regularly in mineral-rich saliva in order to naturally repair tooth defects and weaknesses. Xylitol stimulates mineral-rich saliva to flow into the mouth.[12] By eating a little xylitol regularly, natural tooth healing is encouraged; the more often you eat xylitol, the more healing occurs. Mineral-rich saliva in this way can reverse dental damage and help naturally rebuild and heal cavities without traditional dental treatments. For this reason, although the antibacterial properties of xylitol will occur no matter how it is consumed, I suggest ending every meal, snack, or drink with about one gram of xylitol: either coated on chewing gum, as a breath mint, or eaten directly off a spoon.

Xylitol gum and xylitol mints come in many flavors and textures, and taste as good, or better than, any other gum or breath mint. The difference is that by eating xylitol you change the entire biochemistry of your mouth and help to naturally clean your teeth from a biological point of view while also stimulating natural repair of any damaged or weak areas. Xylitol provides an easy and inexpensive way that can help anyone build strength into their teeth and protect them from wear, cavities, sensitivity, and gum disease.[13]

Xylitol is the perfect partner in any protective dental program. A simple daily routine eating 6 to 10 grams of xylitol can help build the strength of teeth and stop them chipping, wearing down, or breaking. People who eat xylitol notice results quickly, as their teeth become smoother and healthier. What a simple and delicious way to change your dental future!

REPAIRING EARLY CAVITIES: A TRUE STORY

This real-life story is about some young patients of mine who almost wrecked their teeth during a summer-long camping trip. Before the start of their new school year, three teenage boys came to my dental office for their scheduled checkups. Tooth care had obviously been forgotten throughout the summer, and the teenagers admitted to consuming quantities of soda and other damaging drinks and foods throughout their trip. Summer heat and dehydration from their active lifestyles had put the boys at increased risk for cavities. Two of them suffered from allergies, so they each breathed through their mouth, and this put their teeth at even more risk. As we have talked about in earlier chapters, acidity and dry mouth are the two primary factors that lead to weakened teeth and cavities.

I looked at their teeth, and it was apparent that all the molars had been damaged. The middle grooves of each permanent tooth—the first and second molars on both sides of the mouth in the upper and lower jaws—had started to decay. All these teeth had early cavities, a total of eight potential fillings for each boy.

I talked with their mother about the options available. Of course, I could easily put fillings in twenty-four teeth. Alternatively, this family could go home and start a program to rebuild these teeth naturally and replace minerals in the damaged enamel. The most important part of this choice would be taking the situation seriously, since the cavities could progress if the teens did not follow directions.

I explained to this family how remineralization could give the boys the chance to avoid fillings and hopefully have perfect teeth for life. The three were instructed simply to rinse at least twice a day with a dilute fluoride mouthwash and to snack regularly on xylitol-containing gum or mints. Although the outcome was successful, today I would likely suggest the additional use of fluoride varnish to help stimulate remineralization in conjunction with the other products.

On the other hand I have a less cheerful story of a young college student who was told by her dentist she required fifteen fillings. The new lesions had been noticed on X-ray examination during her summer vacation. The filling appointment was scheduled for her winter break. The young college student attended one of my seminars and discovered how xylitol and fluoride can repair weak enamel. This student worked hard for two months to try to repair her tooth damage. Although both her dentist and hygienist noticed great improvement in her teeth and oral health, the fifteen cavities were promptly filled. Although insurance coverage may have been involved in the decision, it seems sad that new X-rays were not taken to see if remineralization was occurring. Any sign of remineralization could have given this patient an opportunity to continue natural healing and a chance to avoid fillings completely.

Acceptance among Dental Professionals

In universities and research institutions in the United States and else-where in the world, many scientists and researchers are familiar with the healing and protective powers of xylitol and the studies showing its effectiveness. For years these people have tried unsuccessfully to disseminate information about the benefits of xylitol to their peers in private practice.

The U.S. military has understood the benefits that xylitol offers; around 2001, it instigated a program called "Look for Xylitol First" to put xylitol chewing gum into packed meals issued to the troops.[14] Soldiers are also advised to check the ingredients in any chewing gum they buy to make sure that xylitol is the number-one ingredient in the gum—and preferably the only sweetener used. The military became concerned about an increase in cavities that occurred when the troops began fighting in desert conditions, where their mouths became dry and unprotected and oral care was difficult or impossible. In 2008, the Association of Dental Hygienists in Arizona adopted xylitol as a preventive method of care; this also happened in Hawaii the follow-ing year.

Michigan, Ohio, and Arizona have been developing programs to introduce mothers and pre-kindergarten children to xylitol, and in Utah some schools have been teaching the use of xylitol for preven-tive dental care. The main surprise is that so few people in the United States are familiar with xylitol and its dental benefits. In every pro-gram and study, participants appear to enjoy the taste of 100 percent xylitol, and it has been shown to be extremely well tolerated by chil-dren and adults.

Unfortunately, throughout much of the country people are con-fused about the difference between xylitol and other sugar alcohols, such as sorbitol and mannitol. Many dentists in general practice clas-sify them together under one umbrella, incorrectly believing that they are all the same. This problem has been aggravated recently by the

ADA's endorsement of a mainly sorbitol-containing chewing gum. Because of the confusion, do not blame your dentist if he or she has overlooked xylitol as a proven method for protecting teeth. Hygienists have recently begun to discuss xylitol in many of their journals and meetings, but other U.S. dental organizations have issued little, if any, encouragement for the use of xylitol.

Besides being a dentist, my husband and I own a restaurant in upstate New York. My passion for dental health led me to install a xylitol-dispensing machine in the kitchen of this restaurant many years ago. I was concerned about the oral health of our many employees because bakery and restaurant staff are noted for having poor oral health. In the environment of a bakery or restaurant there is frequent snacking on sugar, drinking soda on demand, and using breath mints, all of which create a high risk for cavities and dental problems. Even though I knew about the effectiveness of xylitol, I was stunned and amazed to observe firsthand the dramatic improvements we all noticed over the years. The employees who visited dentists regularly were able to bring back reports of how shocked their health professionals were by the improvements in their oral health.

Since then, I have been looking more closely for endorsement of xylitol by the ADA or other organizations. Even though I've found a lot of information on the Internet—including research since the 1970s enumerating the benefits of xylitol—when I typed the word "xylitol" into the search box on the ADA's Research Foundation website in 2002, to my surprise and amusement, a window popped up asking if I meant "Tylenol"! Xylitol was not even in their database. No wonder so many dentists remain unaware of this product and its health benefits.

Dr. Catherine Hayes, an associate professor in the Department of Oral Health Policy and Epidemiology at the Harvard School of Dental Medicine, holds a doctorate in epidemiology and is also a diplomat in public health dentistry. At the turn of the twenty-first century, she participated in a large program that included many well-known scientists, researchers, and dentists from a number of countries and fields of study. Dr. Hayes's group reviewed fourteen studies on the dental effects of eating xylitol and sorbitol that had been published between 1966 and 2000.[15] The latter did not have any long-term effects in reducing tooth decay in children, but evidence overwhelmingly and consistently confirmed that xylitol could be used to control cavities and that it provided strong protection for teeth by removing harmful mouth bacteria.

In her presentation in 2001 to the National Institute of Dental and Craniofacial Research conference in Bethesda, Maryland, Dr. Hayes even went so far as to say that it would be unethical to deprive people of the benefits of xylitol. She concluded her report by saying that "xylitol can significantly decrease the incidence of dental caries."

Ways to Eat Xylitol

Xylitol tastes so good that making it a part of your daily dietary routine is easy. You can eat it as candy, chew it as gum, or use it as a breath mint or spray. Granular xylitol can be made into a solution to wipe or brush onto the teeth of babies, the elderly, or bedridden patients. Some people, especially special-needs patients, may find it easiest to consume xylitol in baked goods, such as puddings and custards, or sprinkled onto foods or into drinks. You need approximately two teaspoons of xylitol each day.

In our restaurant we provide breath mints for patrons to eat after meals as well as individual packets of xylitol at each table for use as a beverage sweetener. Our pastry kitchen experiments with xylitol in its granular form to sweeten cheesecakes, banana and zucchini breads, and other pastries, for instance, to make healthier desserts, especially for guests on a diabetic regimen.

Xylitol was first used as a diabetic sugar more than a hundred years ago. It is gently absorbed by the body and has a low glycemic index. The only setback to baking with xylitol is that it cannot be caramelized, and because it has antifungal properties, it inactivates yeast.

Karen Edwards is a nutritionist and xylitol advocate who has compiled recipes into a book called *Sweeten Your Life the Xylitol Way.* Karen has been working with xylitol for years and has developed a line of chocolate dessert sauces that are available on the Internet as products of Karen's Kitchen.

The structure of xylitol is different from other so-called *sugar alcohols.* In contrast to sorbitol, maltitol, and mannitol, xylitol is in fact well tolerated, and about 15 grams of xylitol is produced naturally in our bodies every day. People who suddenly eat large quantities or replace all the sugar in their diet with xylitol may notice a mild laxative effect at first, because xylitol behaves as a fiber in the diet. But this reaction should not be compared to the bloating and gas after eating even tiny amounts of sorbitol. To avoid any changes from consuming large doses of xylitol, slowly increase the amount you add into your diet.[16] Those who wish to consume large quantities of xylitol regularly can comfortably eat around a hundred grams—about a quarter of a pound—a day, if desired![17]

The only warning for xylitol is that it should not be given to pets and particularly not to dogs. There are many human foods that are not suggested for dogs—grapes, chocolate, and raisins, to name a few. Xylitol is another of these foods; it's better kept away from them.

XYLITOL AFTER MEALS

Many foods take away acidity, but xylitol is one of the most convenient, and it is especially healing for teeth because of its other attributes. Xylitol stimulates a rapid flow of mineral-rich saliva into the mouth, which quickly raises the pH and bathes teeth in healing minerals. Xylitol makes the mouth instantly alkaline, raising the pH to between pH 7.5 and 8.0, which is healthy and safe for teeth. At that alkaline pH, minerals go into teeth and repair weakened areas. Within six months, eating a little xylitol after meals can help anyone with sensitive or weak enamel start to have teeth feel comfortable again. Remember the young Turkish woman who ate lemons and in doing so damaged her teeth? She was able to eat ice cream and drink cold summer beverages without pain or sensitivity within four months of making these simple changes.

This simple product, which has been ignored and discounted in this country for more than thirty years, may be the key to protecting your teeth by yourself. Xylitol will not only help you fight dental disease and the formation of cavities but also may reduce your need for cleanings, sealants, and other treatments at the dentist. For those who do not want to consume xylitol, studies show it is also effective as a mouth rinse or as an ingredient in toothpaste. A Costa Rican study among 2,630 schoolchildren, for example, showed benefits when xylitol was brushed onto teeth twice a day for three years.[18] The problem with toothpaste, however, is the level of abrasiveness, and there may be concerns about other ingredients in the pastes. Those who follow my recommended regimen (outlined in detail in the next chapter) will notice it does not include xylitol-containing toothpaste at this time.

Success Story with Xylitol

Recently I explained to a retired dentist friend of mine and his wife about the way I teach people how to avoid cavities and gum disease with home remedies. The dentist's wife asked if I would tell her the secret, because her teeth were falling apart. Here was a wonderful dentist, an expert in his field, who could not protect his own wife from the disease that was destroying her teeth. I explained how xylitol and simple mouth rinses work in harmony to strengthen teeth. I was impressed by the interest they showed in a new method for improving dental health.

Some weeks later, they told me about the positive effects they had noticed. Those same results have been repeated over and over, and people are amazed at the immediate benefits they feel and see. They cannot believe that something so easy and simple could be so different and effective. People often call me after their dental visits, excited to tell me how much praise they have received and the new level of excellence they have reached with their oral health.

If you are searching for results like these, perhaps it is time to try using xylitol as part of your dental health regimen. Such a simple change may turn the tide, especially people who have difficulty with flossing or who have difficulty taking adequate care of their teeth.

PART SIX

A System for Healthy Teeth

Better put a strong fence round the top of the cliff than an ambulance down in the valley.

—Joseph Malins, "A Fence or an Ambulance" (1895)

Dr. Ellie's Complete Mouth Care System
"A recipe" for adult oral care

For product details and where to purchase these items visit: www.CleanWhiteTeeth.com

You will need:

- A bottle pH balanced, chlorine dioxide rinse
- A new or clean toothbrush
- A tube of Crest® Regular toothpaste
- A bottle antiseptic rinse
- A bottle 0.05% sodium fluoride anticavity rinse
- A small cup for brush storage and toothbrush disinfection
- One or more sources for 100 percent xylitol (no sorbitol!) – Mix and match: mints, gum, wipes, spray, granules etc.
- Optional, pH testing paper.

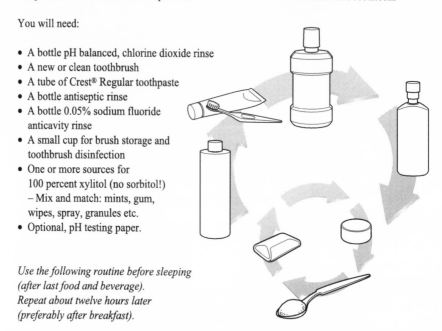

Use the following routine before sleeping (after last food and beverage). Repeat about twelve hours later (preferably after breakfast).

1. Enhance tooth cleaning by using the chlorine dioxide rinse, *before* brushing
2. Brush your gum margin and teeth with a small amount of toothpaste
3. Disinfect all tooth surfaces with the antiseptic rinse, used as "liquid floss"
4. Strengthen, beautify, heal and protect your teeth with the fluoride anticavity rinse
5. Don't re-infect your mouth – disinfect your toothbrush *daily* and store safely.

Use these specific products, exactly in this order, following directions! Like baking a cake, ingredient substitution or changes in method will affect the outcome.

Between these rinsing routines (day or night):

To promote ultimate oral health, expose your teeth to a minimum of 6.5 -10 grams of xylitol each day. This can be in any form: mints, gum, granular etc. Chose a form or forms that work with your lifestyle. For maximum benefit, plan at least 3-5 xylitol exposures each day. Enjoy xylitol after meals, snacks and beverages and whenever your mouth is dry.

For more about prevention and new advances in dentistry, visit: www.cleanwhiteteeth.com *and* AskDrEllie.blogspot.com

CHAPTER THIRTEEN

The Complete Mouth Care System for Adults

I am fortunate to have practiced as both a pediatric and a geriatric dentist, which has allowed me to see the developing teeth of babies, the erupting teeth of children, and the dental challenges for adults of all ages. It often amuses friends to hear how I would travel across Rochester to work in the morning as a pediatric dentist and in the afternoon as a dentist for a senior assisted-living center.

I studied the science of cavities and gum disease as a particular interest, and I used the information to understand the conditions I saw in patients' mouths—patients ranging in age from birth to more than a hundred years old. There were people with healthy teeth who never flossed. There were paranoid tooth flossers with damaged, cavity-laden teeth and eroded gums. Some small children had lost more teeth than some of the ninety-year-olds. I was gradually able to see more clearly why some people enjoyed strong teeth and why it was so difficult for others, no matter how hard they tried, to protect themselves from dental damage.

To find the cause of my patients' dental problems, I always asked a lot of questions. Gradually I discovered that there were similarities and plausible reasons why some teeth became damaged and others did not. Little by little, I collected the information until a clear picture emerged. I asked questions that traced more than just sugar-eating habits. I believed that the problem had to do with the chemistry of the drinks and snacks that people consumed and when they were consumed. I questioned patients with good teeth and beautiful smiles just as much as I questioned those with bad teeth and bad breath. I tried to find the differences in the chemistry of their diets, and more about their food and drink habits, searching to find missing pieces of the puzzle. It slowly became obvious that acidity damaged teeth, and that certain alkaline foods and drinks protected teeth. Even more obvious was the fact that anything damaging was more destructive in a dry mouth. Even the design of bathrooms and how toothbrushes were cleaned and stored became important factors in the quest for oral health.

Your Risk for Dental Disease

John Featherstone is a scientist who worked for many years in the Craniofacial and Mesenchymal Biology Department at the University of California–San Francisco, studying the prevention of dental decay.[1] He describes your risk for dental disease as similar to the risk you would take if riding a motorcycle. At low speeds your risk is less, so you can worry less. At high speeds, your risk is greater, so you need to be more careful if you want to avoid being hurt. People with low risk for dental problems can be more relaxed than those with mouth conditions that put them in the higher-risk group.

It is important to evaluate your personal risk for dental disease. Risk depends on two important factors: mouth acidity and dry mouth. If you have both these problems, you need to take great care if you wish to protect your teeth. The good news is that even those at high risk can use my simple program of protective foods and oral care to control dental problems. Those at greatest risk simply need to take advantage of the system to build strength into their teeth and make sure to regularly protect them.

It seems obvious that if nature is unable to protect your teeth, this job must become yours. Until the time that the surface of your tooth breaks, simple home care can rebuild minerals into tooth enamel and repair any weakness. Softened teeth can be rebuilt, and xylitol has qualities that make your mouth healthier, your teeth less sensitive, and your bite stronger again. Remineralization is the reversal of dental damage, and constantly remineralizing teeth will prevent future problems, even for those in the high-risk category. Strengthening teeth daily is your insurance against soft teeth, wear, breakage, and cavities.

Dr. Ellie's Complete Mouth Care System

This system can help you build density and strength into your teeth, even if you have acidic saliva or you stress your teeth or you have a tooth-grinding habit.

Regular twice-daily use of my complete routine helps people with adult teeth achieve dental health improvement surprisingly quickly. Within weeks, most people find their dental health improving with all the enjoyable results: bad breath fades away, bleeding gums start to heal, and rough teeth feel shiny and smooth. People often write or e-mail me telling of their new sensations, describing their experiences, and delighting in having *happy* teeth for the first time in years.

People with good teeth find the program enhances and safeguards them. Shiny teeth become shinier, healthy gums look better, and teeth feel cleaner. These changes will be obvious to you, and eventually others will notice them. When you have been on the preventive program for a year, you will fully appreciate the change that has occurred. You will see how you have become empowered to protect and strengthen your teeth, all by yourself. You will be able to relax and enjoy your newfound confidence over your dental health.

If you begin with poor oral health you will see dramatic improvements quickly. Bleeding gums will heal and plaque will start to shrink away and stop forming. This is the perfect time to visit your dentist and enjoy a cleaning, to remove the debris of dead plaque and get you off to a nice clean start! When you return from this visit continue with the complete program and at the next six-month visit you should receive the accolades you have always wished to hear from your health professionals. You may decide to explain your improvements, but be aware many dentists will not believe that such a simple system could result in such great improvements. Mostly I suggest keeping the secret to yourself for at least one year; by then your hygienist will demand to know what it is you are doing that makes your teeth so healthy!

If you do not have a cleaning within a couple of months of starting the complete system, the sudden improvement in your oral health may result in a thin band of stain forming around the edges of your teeth, at the gum line. This staining is not a problem, is not permanent, and is not at all unhealthy. This stain is dead plaque debris that has shriveled up and formed a hair-like deposit around the edge of your teeth. One cleaning at the dentist will remove this band of debris and leave your teeth ready for a beautiful new future of healthier, cleaner, and ever-stronger teeth.

Years of experience have convinced me that the majority of people do not have enough respect for their teeth or their tooth enamel. People choose toothbrushes without concern for their quality and toothpaste without scrutiny of the ingredients. Many oral care products are useless; some actually make cleaning teeth more difficult; and a few are outright damaging. There is an art to brushing teeth and an important chemistry between pastes and rinses that must be balanced and appropriate for dental health.

If you use an abrasive toothpaste or one that contains damaging chemicals, you may be weakening your teeth instead of cleaning them. Many mouth rinses are just flavored waters and offer no help at all. Even useful antibacterial mouth rinses can leave your mouth acidic or dry because of the solvents they contain. Rinses can weaken your teeth or, far worse, promote the growth of harmful acid-producing bacteria while you sleep.

I recommend following a complete mouth care system using a particular variety of mouth rinses that are readily available and relatively inexpensive. My main warning is that you must select the products carefully, and if you want the results I describe, then you must use them in this very specific sequence. Adding or subtracting products or substituting other products, even generic substitutions, alters the chemical balance among the ingredients in the system. Using the products in a different sequence, even if they are the exact products, will change the outcome and may reduce the effectiveness of the system. The chemistry and biology of the sequence is exact. Each product has been selected for more than one reason, to be used at a particular time in the sequence, and needs to be used in the prescribed way. I will explain the process in detail and how the products work together. Use the rinsing and brushing system at least twice a day (three times a day, if you like), but most especially before going to bed.

STEP 1: CLEANING PRERINSE

People are surprised that I recommend rinsing the mouth *before* brushing teeth, and the reason may surprise you. A large percentage of adults have acidic saliva or drink acidic drinks just before brushing their teeth. Their teeth will therefore already be acid softened as they start brushing. Acid-softened teeth are easily abraded, especially by a toothbrush coated with toothpaste. Poorly designed brushes, stiff or hard bristles, or an abrasive toothpaste make this problem worse. The teeth most easily damaged will be the first ones hit with the toothpaste, often on the side of your front teeth, opposite the hand that grips the toothbrush.

Some people consume acidic beverages before bed. Beer, wine, soda, or citrus drinks can soften the enamel of your teeth right before you brush them. For this reason it makes sense for everyone to rinse with an acid-neutral rinse, or at least acid-neutral water (check the pH of the water!), before toothbrushing.

I suggest using a stabilized chlorine-dioxide mouth rinse called Closys in the United States (Retardex in the United Kingdom) for a prerinse. This kind of rinse is extremely gentle on the delicate mouth tissues and yet actively removes some kinds of harmful mouth bacteria. This rinse is particularly useful for removing the kind of bacteria that are found in gum pockets around your teeth. Regular use of this rinse helps you to combat pocketing and gum disease. This mouth rinse also breaks down food particles and removes unpleasant breath odor that often contains bad-smelling sulfur.

A chlorine-dioxide rinse is most effective if it is unflavored. The colorless and tasteless liquid may be boring, but users quickly notice its effects. Rinse before brushing using a routine that allows the back teeth to be bathed in the rinse. The area around the back molar teeth is where gum disease usually starts. This rinse is also a good choice for use in an irrigating device such as a Waterpik or water jet for cleaning your teeth. Personally I find this equipment messy and difficult to use, but some of my patients have very positive opinions about it and show great results using it.

STEP 2: TOOTHBRUSHING

I may not talk much about flossing, but I am a fanatic about good toothbrushing. In my office I have always taken part in teaching patients how to brush their teeth effectively. I usually stand behind them, giving my patients a mirror to hold so they can watch me while I brush their teeth. In this way, patients not only feel the benefits of good brushing but also see how it is achieved. Good toothbrushing is especially important for the health of your gums. Use a method that reaches all areas of your mouth, specifically the junction where teeth and gums meet. It is important to choose and maintain a toothbrush that achieves this goal. Select a brush for its effectiveness, but even more important, keep it sanitary and clean! If you use an infected toothbrush, you risk introducing new bacteria and new problems into your mouth.

People often ask if an electric brush is more effective than a manual one. The answer to this question depends on several factors. Do you take an active interest in brushing your teeth? Are you willing to put in the time to brush as thoroughly yourself as an electric brush can? Some people like an electric brush swirling around in their mouths, whereas other people find the sensation nauseating. Disinterested or disabled people will most likely do a better job with an electric brush, but a conscientiously used and well-designed manual brush has been shown in many studies to work as well as any electric brush currently available.

Choosing a Brush

I decided to try an experiment with the staff who work at our restaurant. I purchased a selection of the most commonly available toothbrushes. The waiters and kitchen staff each took two different types and tested them; they reported back on the one they preferred. By the end of our lengthy experiment, we had tried almost 100 different brushes. It finally came down to a choice between two designs. From this selection we chose one brush and arranged with a manufacturer to have the style produced as the Zellies toothbrush. It may not have been the most scientific method of toothbrush evaluation, but most people love Zellies toothbrushes and recommend them to their family and friends. The restaurant employees regard Zellies as exceptionally good stocking stuffers for holiday times. Some patrons at the restaurant have enjoyed a pre-dinner cocktail while simultaneously ordering mouth rinse, Zellies xylitol mints, and a toothbrush from the bartender. In reality, most of the brushes are ordered online from the www.Zellies.com website, but certain stores also sell them. A list of these stores is on the website.

Most people choose a brush that is too big for their mouths or that has too large or long a head. In general, a toothbrush head should be less than one inch in length and should have a handle that allows a firm grasp. The bristles must have rounded ends to avoid damaging the gums. You might think that the more bristles a brush has, the better. In fact, a big brush is more difficult to maneuver around the limited space in your mouth, specifically the upper outside and lower inside areas of your molar teeth. On the other hand, a brush with too few bristles will take too long or possibly never do the job properly.

Many people with poor teeth exhibit gag-reflex problems, and every toothbrush seems too big for them. I suggest looking for "caretaker" brushes with small heads and longer handles, found by searching the Internet. Angled heads, raised bristles, oscillating tufts, and handles that change colors—toothbrushes come in all shapes, colors, and sizes, each promising to perform better than the rest. No scientific evidence that I am aware of shows that any one type of toothbrush design is better than another. The only thing that matters is that you brush effectively. I am sure that your hygienist will be delighted if you ask for a demonstration at your next visit!

The goal is to brush actively around the gums at the junction where they meet the teeth. I call this gum brushing, rather than toothbrushing. It is important that the bristles do not damage your gums, so they must not be too hard or too stiff. The idea is to massage and clean the gums. Softer and more giving bristles allow you to brush your gums more easily and a lot more safely.

Cleaning and Storing a Brush

Although people have begun to realize the hazards of using old, infected toothbrushes, reports still indicate that the average American does not know how to clean a toothbrush and only replaces it once or twice a year. I also suggest that patients remember to buy a new brush to take on vacation and throw it away or disinfect it well on their return. Brushes stored wet in bags can become a real dental hazard.

When I started looking at toothbrushes under a microscope, I began to suggest a far more rigorous routine for toothbrush cleaning and replacement. Brushes should be cleaned *daily*, using an antibacterial or other sanitizing method. Toothbrushes can be cleaned by swishing the bristles of the brush in ½oz undiluted antibacterial rinse (Listerine) for 30 seconds. Rinse away the disinfecting liquids under running tap water. Store the brush head up, in a cup, allowing the bristles to air dry completely between each use. If your storage conditions are damp or wet, mold or bacteria will grow easily on your brush, even under a cover or in a bag. Any infection in your mouth or on your gums can be transferred to your toothbrush bristles, and using an infected brush will replant these bacteria into your mouth at each use.

Storing your brush close to another one allows transfer of bacteria from one brush to another. This fact is very important if you are trying to eliminate cavity-producing or gum-disease bacteria from your mouth. It is also of great concern in schools and daycare centers, where infected brushes can transfer harmful germs from one child's mouth to another. Avoid sharing brushes whenever possible, and remember that wrapping brushes in plastic or storing them in plastic bags is never recommended, unless they have first been disinfected as described above. The makers of the UV sterilizers for toothbrushes are now making small portable units for traveling toothbrushes, and the units seem to work well. Depending on their bathroom conditions, some families may be able to keep their toothbrushes cleaner by storing them in a kitchen area.

Choosing a Toothpaste

Toothpaste is a huge industry. Most people have been affected by the power of advertising and select pastes they hope will cure any dental problems and improve their smile.

Many people are affected by the antibacterial chemicals and tartar-control ingredients contained in toothpastes. Some of these chemicals offer bacterial protection, but they may sensitize the skin of the mouth and cause sores or ulceration. Patients rarely associate mouth ulceration with their toothpaste. If you have a history of mouth soreness, discontinue your toothpaste and see if the ulcers clear up.

My suggestion would be to use as few chemicals as possible in your mouth! Find old-fashioned, boring toothpastes that will keep you safe and better protected!

Toothpaste was used as early as the fourth century. Ancient Egyptian manuscripts describe a paste made from salt, pepper, mint, and the iris flower. Other records tell of pastes and powders made from eggshells and animal hooves. Modern toothpastes were developed in the early 1800s and originally were dispensed from a jar. It was not until the late 1800s that a special toothpaste, Dr. Sheffield's Crème Dentifrice, was first put into a collapsible tube. Early toothpaste contained ingredients such as myrrh, sage, peppermint, strawberry, and eucalyptus.

Today many of these same ingredients are used in herbal pastes (even iris flower). Most pastes contain dicalcium phosphate dehydrate as an abrasive to clean teeth. Abrasive toothpaste, often used for tartar control, can cause sensitivity and may actually weaken teeth. Baking soda is a popular choice, but with prolonged use it can also cause gum irritation. As I pointed out earlier, some antibacterial ingredients and whitening products may even be classified as co-carcinogens, capable of triggering cancer in cancer-prone patients when used repeatedly over time.

I suggest a paste that is gentle and not too abrasive, with as few additives as possible. I prefer pastes that were formulated before the advent of the whitening craze, and I recommend the original Crest Regular Cavity Protection toothpaste with no extras. This paste is sufficiently cleansing without being too abrasive. It contains sodium fluoride to strengthen teeth and fits perfectly into the system of care that I recommend. Do not expect your toothpaste to be a one-stop shop for all your dental needs. Look for the ADA seal of approval, which indicates that the association has tested the product for safety and effectiveness. Even if you see the seal of acceptance, do not take your eye off the list of ingredients! It is technically possible to clean your teeth effectively without any toothpaste, or you could use a solution of xylitol (half a teaspoon stirred in two ounces of water), a good option for anyone with a very dry mouth or who finds regular toothpaste too strong in taste. Alternatively, using a little fluoride mouth rinse (ACT) on your toothbrush is another suggestion for someone with a delicate mouth and damaged teeth.

STEP 3: RINSE (TWICE) AFTER BRUSHING

I recommend a sequence of two more mouth rinses after you've brushed your teeth. Rinses have various chemistries and therefore different effects. My system uses rinses that reduce the chance of developing gum disease while building the strength of your teeth. One rinse follows the other. Together these mouth rinses leave your teeth feeling amazingly clean, and over time, you will notice remarkable benefits.

An antiseptic rinse is used first to rinse toothpaste off your teeth and kill immature plaque germs. The biggest problem with most antiseptic mouth rinses is that they are usually highly acidic. If an acidic rinse remains on your teeth, it has the potential to soften tooth enamel and cause it to become weak and brittle. The most effective rinses also contain a high percentage of alcohol, which can dry the mouth. Dry and acidic conditions create the perfect breeding ground for harmful mouth bacteria, which themselves create more mouth acidity. Leaving an acidic rinse on your teeth can potentially create conditions that lead to gum irritation and infection, softened teeth, cavities, and even bad breath.

The problem may be particularly frustrating for people who have a dry mouth or previously acid-damaged teeth. These people find acidic antibacterial rinses make their tooth enamel so soft it can be worn down by nighttime tooth clenching and grinding. Senior citizens frequently use antibacterial rinses for their dental problems, but without enough moisture to dilute and wash away the acidity of the antiseptic rinses, damage can result. Who would think that a mouthwash might actually promote dental problems?

I suggest using an antiseptic rinse *followed immediately* by a protective rinse, just as in skin care people are always advised to follow the toner with a moisturizer. Rinse your mouth thoroughly with an antiseptic, and as soon as you spit it out, use a protective rinse. Antiseptic rinses can feel harsh, but use them quickly or even dilute them with warm water, if necessary.

Antiseptic Rinse

Listerine was the first mouth rinse to receive the ADA seal of acceptance for helping control the gum inflammation called *gingivitis*. The main ingredients in Listerine are menthol, thymol, and eucalyptus oil. Thymol, one of the most effective of the essential oils, is a powerful germicide and fungicide. Eucalyptus is produced from the blue gum tree, a plant native to Australia.

Recent testing confirms the effectiveness of Listerine in removing plaque from teeth and shows that rinsing twice a day is as effective for removing plaque as flossing once a day. Listerine exerts its antibacterial effect mainly on immature bacteria, so rinsing every twelve hours is important. The bonus of Listerine is that rinsing reaches everywhere in the mouth whereas only about 25 percent of the mouth is cleaned by flossing and brushing.

Some people worry about the amount of ethyl alcohol in the product, but many studies by the ADA and the National Cancer Institute show this ingredient to be completely safe. Another concern raised in this age of the overuse of antibiotics is whether a tolerance or resistance would be created by regular use. It is comforting to read the studies and find that the essential oils contained in Listerine do not result in such resistance complications. Even today, with all the alternatives available, Listerine appears to be one of the oldest yet most effective mouth rinses available.

When selecting from the array of Listerine flavor choices, look for the original formula or a taste you can tolerate. Avoid rinses that are advertised for plaque control, whitening, or have other features that are unnecessary. Make sure you purchase a product that has the ADA seal on the bottle; the genuine original may be the best. If necessary, rinse quickly or dilute the rinse to your own tolerance level. Most important of all, do not leave the rinse on your teeth when you go to bed! Listerine is acidic and could potentially be a problem, so be sure to wash it off your teeth with a final protective rinse to complete the suggested system.

Protective Rinse

For shiny, strong, and healthy teeth I recommend a dilute fluoride finishing rinse to protect your teeth at the conclusion of the system. Although I filter fluoride out of my drinking water, I am a proponent of using a 0.05 percent sodium fluoride rinse called ACT anticavity rinse as part of my system of adult oral care, especially before sleeping. It is especially important if you have damaged or weak teeth, lack natural protection (dry mouth), or are middle-aged or older (at high risk for dental disease and damage).

A fluoride rinse will have a strengthening effect on tooth enamel, rebuilding it to an extra-hard strength. The volume of fluoride rinse in your mouth is not important; more important is how long the rinse remains in contact with your teeth. Keep the fluoride rinse in your mouth as long as possible and preferably make it the last thing you do before going to bed so that a thin film of residue stays on your teeth while you are sleeping. The longer you keep fluoride on the outside of your teeth, the more it will strengthen your tooth enamel.

I have been asked whether fluoride rinsing is desirable if you live in a fluoridated area. The answer depends on the state of your teeth. If you need help for soft, damaged, or decayed teeth, rinsing with fluoride will improve their strength and condition. If your teeth are sensitive, if they flake or have fillings, a fluoride rinse will protect them and build strength into surrounding enamel. Fluoride rinsing is a good choice for a final rinse if you have any silver or white fillings in your mouth since it will help maintain enamel strength and help you avoid repairs. Depending on the kind of fillings that you have, this can save you from possible exposure to mercury and its very negative consequences. For preventive reasons, fluoride rinsing is healthier than having disease in your mouth, and the benefits make it worthy of adding to your daily oral care routine.

For anyone who refuses to put fluoride into his or her mouth, the next best rinse would be one containing all natural ingredients and xylitol.

How This Dental Care System Helps Women

I have always believed, based on my clinical experience, that women's dental problems not only start at a younger age but also are different from those experienced by men. I have noticed that natural protection for women's teeth begins to disappear as they enter their middle to late thirties. Initial changes in teeth are seen as sensitivity along the gum margin. Visually this is seen as a groove in the enamel, high up the tooth at the gum margin, most often on upper-back molar teeth. The appearance is of a channel, almost as if the tooth enamel has been worn away by bad toothbrushing, and the patient is often told that gum recession has occurred.

There are many philosophies about the cause of this sensitive groove, but I believe enamel flakes chip away from the sides of the tooth surface at places where the tooth enamel is thin and unsupported. Tooth enamel is most vulnerable where teeth bend and flex; for example, at the point where the crown of the tooth becomes the soft cement of the root surface. The damaged area can be extremely sensitive to hot and cold, liquids, air, and brushing. Sometimes the pain of cold or touch will last for some time, which can make brushing the area very painful.

Similar damage usually occurs at the same time in the enamel surrounding fillings. As the sensitive groove becomes painful, old fillings usually start to hurt and fail. Tooth enamel abuts the edge of the fillings in such a way that it leaves a thin enamel flange around each filling. Erosion and chipping are responsible for the groove at the gum line and are also responsible for the breakage of this ledge enamel. As the seal around each filling breaks, liquids from the mouth will penetrate the small gap that opens up and travel underneath the filling.

Fillings rarely solve the sensitivity problem, and the patient most often needs root-canal treatment and removal of the nerves in the affected teeth. Once the root canal has been completed, crowns will be required. Unfortunately, the timing of this will coincide with the onset of gum disease around the back teeth in both the upper and lower jaws. Periodontal surgery will keep the unfortunate patient in the dental chair for repeated and extensive treatments, often leading to tooth loss and implants or dentures.

If mouth acidity and the cause of dental disease are addressed at the first sign of sensitivity, however, the entire sequence of treatment will most likely be prevented.

How This Dental Care System Helps Pregnant Women

A woman is at more risk for gum disease and cavities during pregnancy than at any other time in her life. A number of coincidental factors predispose a pregnant woman to both these conditions. Many women start their pregnancy with hormonal changes that can cause dehydration and nausea. Vomiting exposes dental enamel to gastric acids that weaken tooth enamel. Often the immediate reaction after vomiting is to brush teeth using toothpaste, but cleaning acid-softened teeth with toothpaste, which is abrasive, can rub away the outer tooth-protective layer.

Following an acidic exposure it is important to return the mouth to a neutral, or balanced, nonacidic state before brushing your teeth. An alkaline or balanced mouth rinse, alkaline or neutral nonacidic foods, or alkaline water should achieve balance before toothbrushing starts. It is also important for a pregnant woman to strengthen her tooth enamel after the weakening that is caused by these acid attacks. Toward the end of pregnancy acid reflux may be a problem, especially at night, when the gastric acids have similar weakening effects on tooth enamel.

In the final trimester, the dental situation is further complicated because there is a dramatic change in a mother's saliva. Around the twenty-seventh week of pregnancy, the saliva in the mouth suddenly loses its ability to neutralize acids. This extraordinary condition leaves teeth and gums very vulnerable to damage during the last trimester. Natural protection returns to normal at delivery. It is astonishing to discover how few people, especially women, know about this change and the need for extra dental protection during the last twelve weeks of pregnancy. The reason for the change is not understood, but it makes dental strengthening and healing essential for pregnant women if they are to prevent their teeth from being softened and damaged.

Other dental problems during pregnancy come from changes in diet and routines that reflect a new lifestyle. During pregnancy, eating and drinking patterns may change; some women give up work or change their sleep patterns. Pregnant women may also change the types of foods they eat; they often crave juice or foods that are acidic. Juices such as orange, apple, and grapefruit can soften teeth and damage them enough to result in cavities by the end of the pregnancy. Fruited herbal teas also may be acidic, and despite their beneficial health effects, may harm tooth enamel during a pregnancy. New mothers need to be aware that even healthy food choices can leave the mouth acidic and result in tooth damage. The great news is that by protecting teeth with xylitol you can still enjoy these foods but protect teeth immediately after eating them.

Restless nights can result in snacks during normal sleep time. There is always less natural saliva to wash away harmful liquids from teeth at night, and pregnant women need to know that tooth damage occurs quickly when acidity and dry mouth occur at the same time. Snack food should be as nonacidic, sugar free, and dentally protective as possible, but eating some xylitol before returning to bed is another good option.

A pregnant woman needs to know how to deal with acidity if she is to safely enjoy her snacks and drinks. Eating an alkaline food at the end of a meal or after a drink will balance mouth acidity, leave the saliva alkaline, and protect the teeth. Alkaline foods include nuts, cheese, celery and other raw vegetables, fresh apples, yogurt, bananas, and—of course—xylitol.

Xylitol mints or gum protect teeth after any drink or snack (especially if you are unable to clean your teeth before sleeping) and help to reduce the number of harmful plaque germs. Make informed food and drink choices and eat plenty of foods containing calcium (cheese, yogurt, and peanut butter). Choose nonacidic beverages and water whenever possible or protect your teeth after any acidic drink or snack by eating a xylitol mint or gum.

In addition, pregnant women may devote less time to oral care routines. Whenever short of time or energy for brushing, remember that xylitol can help protect your teeth. Most important, when you use xylitol during pregnancy, you are cleaning your mouth and allowing the colonization of your teeth by healthy, protective bacteria. These are the bacteria you want to pass on to your newborn. The babies of mothers with clean and healthy mouths have less dental disease and around 70 percent fewer cavities than do the children of mothers who have harmful mouth bacteria.

If you are planning a pregnancy, consider your dental health. Research shows that having healthy gums can reduce preterm births by 84 percent. Other studies show that the more gum disease a pregnant woman has, the greater her chance of delivering a low-birth-weight baby. It is especially important to prepare gums and make them healthy *before* becoming pregnant since treatment during pregnancy may not reverse the risk.

A number of cultures teach women that a tooth will be lost for each baby. Over the years many women have found that this old wives' tale appears to be true, because pregnant women develop cavities, bleeding gums, dental pain, and loose teeth during pregnancy. What really happens is that there is a dramatic change in mouth chemistry during pregnancy. The resulting damage validates an incorrect belief that calcium has been pulled out of teeth to supply the baby's bones. In truth, there is a predictable chain of events that can cause serious damage to a woman's teeth by the time her baby is born. The damage can be easily avoided if teeth are properly protected during pregnancy.

How This Dental Care System Helps Men

Dental problems for men appear to occur a decade or so later than acidic damage that affects the teeth of women. Men generally do not seem to be plagued by mouth acidity and do not seem to show the same kinds of tooth damage. Unless they have had a history of gum disease or active tooth decay, most men survive without dental problems until their mid-to-late fifties. The onset of their problems usually occurs when they find their mouths become drier. Dry mouth symptoms are erosion of tooth enamel, wear of teeth and the enamel around fillings (resulting in loss of fillings), gum disease, and bad breath. Someone with acid reflux and a dry mouth will have similar but possibly more serious problems that affect oral health at an alarming rate. Medications that affect liquid balance or have mouth-drying side effects can also precipitate similar dental damage.

Most of these dental problems can be likened to the damage a car engine incurs when the oil level drops too low to lubricate the engine parts. As men age, their mouths become drier, and with a change in muscle tone, their jaw muscles relax. Older men may find they routinely sleep with their mouths open, causing teeth to dry even more. Clenching or grinding dry teeth can wear tooth enamel, which shows up as shortening of the teeth, flattening of the biting surfaces of the teeth, and loosening of fillings as enamel is ground away. Even more damage is done to tooth enamel when porcelain crowns crash against soft and unprotected natural teeth.

In a dry mouth, tooth enamel becomes brittle and prone to cracking and breaking. If the enamel chips around fillings, the seal breaks and allows leakage under the fillings. Leaking fillings become the breeding ground for bacteria that cause disease under fillings and may kill the nerve. All these factors result in the need for replacement fillings, root-canal treatments, and crowns. Some dentists suggest entire mouth rehabilitation, which involves building back the original height of the teeth all around the mouth. This kind of work is expensive and time consuming. Gum disease, both mild and severe, is also a common problem for men by the age of sixty. It is not good for general health, and as we discussed earlier, gum inflammation is linked to high blood pressure, coronary plaque formation, and heart disease.

The daily routine of mouth rinses suggested in this chapter can always be used as a preventive measure, but it becomes especially important for men as they pass middle age, especially for anyone with a dry mouth who notices his teeth becoming worn or chipped, or who takes medications that have a mouth-drying side effect.

How This Dental Care System Helps Seniors and Those with Special Needs

People past retirement age often suffer a combination of damage. As seniors lose their ability to eat regular foods, they often replace normal meals with a more acidic diet consumed in small quantities and at frequent intervals. Our local Veterans Administration hospital reports show that men admitted with good teeth have lost them all by the end of the first year in the hospital.

Medications with mouth-drying side effects relax muscle tone while making the patient drowsy. When a patient sleeps with an open mouth, salivary flow is reduced, and breathing through the mouth further dries the teeth. Liquid diets frequently contain citric acid, which leaches calcium from teeth and creates the perfect environment for dental disease. The result is chipped enamel, tooth breakage, heavy plaque buildup, bad breath, and deterioration of fillings.

Regular consumption of xylitol or the use of a xylitol spray has been shown to improve the health of mouth tissues as well as the health of teeth, so it is useful even for patients who have dentures. Xylitol protects against fungus-caused denture sores in the mouth and the painful cracks caused by fungal infections that develop at the corners of the mouth in the elderly and chronically sick.

People with extremely dry mouths may find mouth rinses with alcohol are too harsh to tolerate. Prerinsing with Closys cleans the mouth tissues and protects against gum disease. It should be followed by toothbrushing with a fluoride or xylitol paste or by brushing with xylitol solution, depending on the tolerance of the patient. For those able to rinse and spit effectively, a final rinse with ACT gives long-lasting protection and increases the enamel's resistance to damage. In some cases the fluoride rinse can be wiped or brushed onto soft or damaged teeth.

Dental treatment may be challenging, difficult, and even frightening or traumatic for those with mental, physical, or developmental disabilities. Crowded teeth may be hard to clean, and many patients dislike the feel of toothpaste or toothbrushes in their mouth. Many developmentally disabled patients have larger-than-normal tongues and high-vaulted and narrow-roofed mouths, all of which make oral care a particular challenge for caretakers. People who are bedridden, in wheelchairs, or in neck braces cannot reach sinks to rinse or spit. If plaque grows thick in these mouths, cavities, gum disease, and even systemic general health implications result. Chronically ill patients often have irreparable dental disease to add to their miseries. Simple solutions can prevent this kind of damage.

Eating xylitol regularly or using xylitol to clean teeth reduces plaque and controls buildup. If chewing gum or eating mints is not an option, use xylitol wipes or mouth spray. A solution of xylitol in water can be wiped on teeth with a sponge or a gauze square to clean them, or the solution can be rinsed around the mouth or brushed onto teeth. It is acceptable to swallow excess solution (which tastes good) if spitting is not possible. Recently, a lozenge (XyliMelts) with an adhesive backing has been developed which can be stuck onto a tooth or placed on an appliance or a feeding tube and allowed to slowly dissolve, without the need to chew or keep it moving in the mouth.

Keep toothbrushes clean at all times to avoid transferring harmful bacteria into the mouth. Some living facilities clean patients' teeth with sponges soaked in lemon juice and glycerin. This treatment is not recommended because it is an acidic solution and offers no protection for teeth. A xylitol solution or xylitol-impregnated tooth wipe, like Spiffies or Floss and Wipe, is a much better option.

Patients in hospital situations often need feeding tubes and mouth appliances that prop the mouth open. These tubes create a drying situation that leaves teeth vulnerable. The longer the debilitated condition or sickness continues, the worse the dental damage is likely to be. The drier the mouth, the less protection for teeth, and in these situations, gum disease often develops quickly. There is now considerable evidence that a relationship exists among poor oral health, the bacteria in the mouth, and bacterial pneumonia. Together, pneumonia and influenza constitute the sixth most common cause of death in the United States and in most developed countries. The bacteria grow on teeth or dentures and then become aspirated (sucked) into the lower airway, where lung infection develops. Recent studies show that controlling plaque and gum infection can reduce or prevent pneumonia in high-risk vulnerable and hospitalized patients.

During the studies, it also became clear that antibiotic treatment increases the chance that harmful bacteria will colonize the patients' teeth. It would appear that antibiotic treatments eliminate the protective plaque bacteria and leave teeth exposed and vulnerable to infection by other bacteria. Healthy, protective plaque forms a layer to defend teeth, but without that layer, teeth are easily infected by other kinds of aggressive bacteria, possibly reaching the patient through toothbrush contamination or contact with hospital staff, other patients, or visitors who have dental disease.

How This Dental Care System Helps Athletes

Surprisingly, the risk profile of an athlete is similar to that of a debilitated patient. The cycle of damage involves the same two elements: an acidic environment and a dry mouth. A dehydrated athlete, such as a runner, will have thick, acid-prone saliva. The dry mouth and lack of saliva leave the athlete at risk for tooth damage.

The consumption of acidic sports drinks sweetened with sugar or glucose will feed harmful acid-producing bacteria. Fruited herbal teas and even juices (such as orange juice) contain citric acid that can cause great damage in a dry mouth. The generalized mouth acidity and buildup of bacteria could cause gingivitis and inflammation of the gums. A dehydrated athlete may be at further risk if acidic or sugary drinks are alternated with sugar or carbohydrate bars.

Lack of saliva reduces the lubrication that normally protects teeth, so teeth are at risk for dental erosion, and they wear quickly when clenched or ground during moments of intense concentration. It is important that athletes take care to use protective programs to super-strengthen their teeth as often as possible. Athletes should also take steps to control dental disease, eliminate harmful bacteria in their mouths, and protect their teeth.

As I discussed in the chapter on food for teeth, sports drinks and protein shakes often contain sorbitol, a low-calorie sweetener that has received FDA safety clearance for use as a sugar substitute in candies, drinks, and confections. When sorbitol is eaten regularly it appears that bacteria in plaque adapt in such a way as to use sorbitol as an energy source for growth. An increased number of potentially harmful bacteria in the mouth may contribute to gum disease. No one wants to encourage harmful plaque bacteria, so it is advisable for people—especially someone with a dehydrated mouth—to avoid drinks and snacks containing sorbitol.

Look for sports meals and drinks that use xylitol, which makes your mouth less hospitable to dangerous germs. Eat xylitol mints or chew xylitol gum before and during exercise, before napping, and whenever you need to clean or protect your teeth. Look for alternative drinks made with xylitol or follow acidic and citric drinks with xylitol mints or gum to bring the mouth back to an alkaline state. Drinking alkaline juices or mineral waters are best from a dental point of view. As mentioned earlier, Evian water and Fiji water are alkaline bottled waters that would be protective of teeth.

Saliva flow is important to protect your teeth, and consuming xylitol stimulates saliva flow and makes the mouth acid neutral.

How This Dental Care System Helps Diabetics

Diabetes mellitus affects an estimated 20 million Americans, and the incidence is increasing each year. The relationship between diabetes and gum disease has been studied for more than fifty years, revealing that diabetes is associated with an increased risk for serious gingivitis and gum disease.

Correspondingly, the presence of gum disease can make the control of diabetes more difficult. Treating gum disease and reducing mouth inflammation both have a positive effect for diabetics. Patients with Type II diabetes who did not have gum infection had six times better glycemic control than those with gum disease.

Diabetics should consider the complete mouth-care system with xylitol if they have been unable to control their dental health with other products. Your doctor should be notified of any dietary changes you make, but xylitol is a safe natural product for diabetics and is easy to eat throughout the day and even during times of sleeplessness at night. Xylitol has a glycemic index of 7.0 and is safe for hypoglycemic patients also. Xylitol may also offer relief and positive benefits to diabetic patients who suffer from acid reflux.

For a schematic diagram of this system see page 162 or visit www.CleanWhiteTeeth.com.

CHAPTER FOURTEEN

The Complete Mouth Care
System for Children

Children who have perfect teeth at eighteen years old (or when all their permanent teeth have erupted) are more likely than others to have perfect teeth for life. Parents have the power to give their children a lifetime of cavity-free teeth, but there are some critical times to take action. The window of opportunity is small. Parents must be aware of the sequence and timing when teeth erupt and will want to allow sufficient time to change the quality of mouth bacteria before new teeth come into the mouth during childhood and adolescence.

Prenatal Care

In a stunning research project a significant benefit for children was seen when mothers ate a few grams of xylitol each day, starting before the birth of her child. Researchers found that the children had healthier teeth and the beneficial effects continued for years, even after the preventive program stopped. If a new mother will eat some xylitol each day during the first year of her baby's life, she will have the opportunity to improve her baby's dental health by up to 80% compared with control groups.

Yet, in 2006, the wife of a friend of mine was about to have a baby, and I described the details of this study to him. I ordered xylitol-containing chewing gum from the same company that made the chewing gum for this research project twenty-five years previously. I gave some of the gum to the expectant couple in the hopes that they would start a preventive program. The young man talked with the mother, who in turn talked with her OB/GYN. The doctor told them he had never heard of this method of dental disease prevention and advised her not to eat the product.

Studies show that the greatest reduction in harmful bacteria comes from eating products sweetened with 100 percent xylitol. Parents who chew xylitol gum or eat xylitol mints each day from the time the baby is born will gradually clean away unhealthy bacteria from their mouths before the eruption of the baby's first tooth. With a little effort, parents can give their baby a great start to dental health.

Infants

Friendly germs and cavity germs fight to live on your child's tooth, and the first one on the tooth wins! If friendly germs are first to reach a new tooth, they will take over, and the child's chance of future cavities can be reduced.

For added protection and to ensure your baby's mouth is healthy before teeth begin to erupt, wipe his or her gums with a 100 percent xylitol wipe such as Spiffies (available on the Internet), or let your baby enjoy xylitol-sweetened water between feedings.

Baby teeth first erupt at around six or seven months of age and continue, a few at a time, until the child is around two years old. Some of the last baby teeth to emerge are baby molars that have wrinkled biting surfaces perfect for chewing and grinding food. There are natural pits and crevices in the biting surfaces where bacteria can quickly become entrenched. If harmful bacteria aggressively populate these areas, any sugar in the diet will feed them. With energy from the sugar, the bacteria reproduce and form acids that cause tooth damage in the depths of the pits and crevices.

The enamel of new molars takes almost a year to become strong enough to resist acid attacks. Pediatric dentists often need to fill cavities in the biting surfaces of new molars before a child's third birthday, before the teeth have even had time to fully mature and harden. Whether a mother is breast-feeding, using formula, or feeding her child solid food, she should worry about the kind of bacteria in these molar crevices and also try to control the acidity and sugar content of drinks and foods, especially when her child has a dry mouth while napping or sleeping.

Because proper cleaning of your baby's teeth is often difficult, make sure your baby is protected at all times by encouraging the growth of healthy bacteria in the mouth both before and during the time that molars erupt. For babies, toothpaste is not necessary. In fact, many children's toothpastes are bad for teeth, because they contain sugar or sorbitol. Use a soft toothbrush dipped in a solution made from an individual packet of granular xylitol dissolved in warm water or a xylitol-containing toothpaste or spread a xylitol gel on the teeth and gums. Baby wipes containing xylitol can also be useful.

BREAST MILK

The art of breast-feeding can be difficult, and the last thing a new mother needs to hear are unfounded concerns that she may be inducing cavities in her baby's teeth. A 1999–2002 National Health and Nutrition Examination Survey provided data that were used by the University of Rochester School of Medicine and Dentistry to evaluate more than 1,500 children between the ages of two and five. They found that neither breast-feeding nor its duration is associated with increased risk of early tooth decay in children (www.ada.org/goto/sciencenews).

Understandably, then, I was dismayed in 2005 to see headlines on the front page of my local paper proclaiming a link between breast-feeding and cavities. I wrote to the paper in protest, explaining my frustration with the way the article had been written. Careful examination revealed that the study was conducted among laboratory animals under unusual conditions. The animals had been prepared for the experiment by having their salivary glands surgically removed. The animals had no natural protection for their teeth. Next, the animals were infected with the most aggressive acid-producing bacteria, a strain that causes the most possible cavities. Breast milk was fed to the animals constantly and, not surprisingly, some cavities developed in the teeth.

The headlines were sensational, but the study did not address reality. The choice of nutrition for a baby should be based on the healthiest option possible. Before teeth erupt into the mouth, there will be no damage to them from any of the liquids selected: formula, cow's milk, or breast milk. The issue occurs *after* teeth are present. Many mothers fear that breast milk has caused problems for their children's teeth. Experiments like the one described in our local paper perpetuate such ideas. I would like, rather, to have seen this article explain that a mother *can control* the kind of bacteria in her baby's mouth. With healthy bacteria in the baby's mouth there will be no acid-producing bacteria. All mothers, including those who are nursing, should try to ensure that there are only protective bacteria on their baby's teeth. This way there will not be conditions to promote tooth decay.

I am sorry to see mothers concerned that breast-feeding could harm their child's teeth. I would counsel mothers to worry more about their own dental health, toothbrush hygiene, the ingredients in teething gels and, where possible, use xylitol-containing products to clean a child's mouth and protect the new teeth.

Baby bottles and sippy cups do not cause tooth decay (see the discussion in chapter 4), but once your baby has teeth, be careful what goes into that baby bottle or sippy cup! Avoid anything acidic: fruit punch, Kool-Aid, or fruit juices (orange, apple, or grape), even if the juices are diluted. Any of these acidic drinks will attack new teeth. Cow's milk is safe, but many brands of infant formula can cause decay. A solution of a few grams of xylitol in warm water is a great alternative. Sweeten cow's milk with xylitol to make a dentally safe sweet drink for baby. Adding half a teaspoon to an eight-ounce baby bottle would be plenty to sweeten the water and yet give dental protection.

Toddlers

It may be useful to explain here how the protective effect of using xylitol occurs. We discussed in chapter 3 that molar grooves were the reservoirs of harmful tooth bacteria in the mouth. We know that eating xylitol for a period of six months can clean the mouth of harmful bacteria and set up the stage for healthy, protective bacteria to populate the mouth. Baby molar teeth erupt at around two years of age, and making sure the mouth is clean of harmful bacteria when new baby teeth erupt will help ensure that the baby molar grooves are filled with only healthy bacteria.

If this window of opportunity is missed there is another one— before permanent molars erupt at six years of age. Changing the kind of mouth bacteria before these teeth enter the mouth will ensure that the reservoir for the permanent teeth contains only healthy mouth bacteria. This is the logic behind the regular use of xylitol in Scandinavian preschool and kindergarten programs.

The ages two to four are also important years in which to establish good dental-care habits, and for many parents, they are some of the most challenging years. Toddlers are very busy little people. They want to do more things on their own, and they love to learn new things. This is the time to establish a regular dental-care routine. Be sure toddlers have their own toothbrushes, and disinfect them regularly.

Encourage your toddlers to brush their teeth. Teach them to brush before bedtime and make it part of their nighttime routine. They will not be brushing thoroughly, so they will need your help. Use a pea-sized amount of a simple fluoride or xylitol toothpaste without tartar control, whiteners, or other additives. If the taste is too strong, use a few drops of a mild-flavored 0.05 percent fluoride (bubble-gum ACT) rinse on the toothbrush.

Teach your toddler how to brush and spit properly. This is also a great time to introduce xylitol gum or mints during the day. Toddlers love candy, and xylitol products are a healthy substitute that protects and strengthens their teeth.

It is good to have new teeth checked with a trained eye that can look for early signs of damage and talk with you about preventive measures. It is never too early to have good professional dental advice, because there are many ways to stop early cavities.

If your child's teeth show signs of damage, do not be alarmed. It takes about a year or more for a cavity to reach a stage that needs a filling, so if you know there are problems, you should have time to try to reverse them. If you find out that your baby has the start of cavities, rethink your baby's diet and try to figure out a reason why the condition is occurring. Simple changes and a little more protection from the culprit foods or drinks may be all you need. Look for an acidic problem, most often juice. As mentioned previously, apple juice appears to be one of the most damaging.

Often you do not have to eliminate or change the habits that have caused the problem, just be aware of what is causing the decay. Protect your baby's teeth from damage by giving him or her some xylitol after the juice. Use xylitol candy or gum, some granular xylitol, or just a drink of xylitol dissolved in water. Fresh apples, vegetables, cheese, or dairy also remove mouth acidity and provide minerals for teeth. The use of protective foods and xylitol protects teeth and may help to repair them. Cutting down slowly on the juice will be helpful, but a protective approach allows you to do it in a pleasant and enjoyable way, without adding stress—or yelling—to your day.

White spots are often the first signs of weakened teeth. The enamel will look dull or feel rough. It is important to protect this enamel, and nothing sharp should be pushed into this tooth to test its hardness. Weak enamel can be hardened and rebuilt to its original strength just by eating xylitol or combined with a little fluoride applied as a varnish by the dentist if he or she is agreeable. If the problem is addressed, teeth can remain strong; even a damaged tooth can last until the permanent one erupts.

Xylitol solution or wipes used on damaged teeth help harden them. At this stage your toddler will usually be napping regularly and may be prone to ear infections and colds. These infections may cause your toddler to breathe through the mouth at nap time, which causes the toddler's mouth to become dry and more prone to cavities, because it will not have the natural protection of saliva.

Encourage your toddler to eat xylitol in some form before nap time or use a xylitol wipe to clean his or her teeth. In chapter 12 you read about the xylitol research that has shown that ear infections can be reduced by up to 40 percent with regular consumption of xylitol each day. Protection occurs because the bacteria in the tubes from the throat into the ears are populated by healthy and protective bacteria, in the same way the mouth bacteria are changed. You can also use a nasal spray on children (or toddlers who will tolerate the experience) to help control the harmful bacteria in the throat and ear tubes.

Young Children

The protective effect of xylitol for children's teeth depends on when it is eaten. Bacteria counts double or triple after eating, so use xylitol after meals and snacks. The most powerful effect in reducing tooth decay occurs when xylitol is eaten regularly for a whole year before a tooth erupts (this gives a 93 percent reduction in cavities). Eating xylitol for a year before the eruption of permanent molars (at five to six years old) gives maximum protection for future adult teeth. After a two-year period of eating xylitol, the protective effect will be seen for many years later.

When a child is between five and six years old, the first molars start to come into the mouth. These molars are important adult teeth and need to last a lifetime. The new teeth have grooves in their biting surfaces. It is important that the grooves be populated with healthy bacteria. Research shows healthy bacteria protect teeth as well as any plastic sealant applied by a dentist and that the effect of natural protection is long-lived.

New teeth are soft and very easily damaged. Because it takes about a year for them to harden, many molars are damaged and have cavities within a year of erupting. A filling at age five can cause lifelong problems, with many repairs and possibly root-canal treatments and crowns. The time to avoid all those future adult visits to the dentist is when your child is between five and twelve years old. Xylitol is here to help you reduce the chance of tooth decay by at least 70 percent!

Zellies mints and gum make it easy for you to give your children the chance for healthier teeth by protecting their teeth from acids, controlling unhealthy bacteria, and helping repair damage to teeth. Your children will love the sweet taste of xylitol. You will love that their teeth are being protected and repaired. Let your child chew a couple of pieces of xylitol gum or eat a couple of xylitol mints after every meal, snack, or drink.

If your child has a dry mouth because of mouth breathing, medications, allergies, or asthma, encourage extra xylitol throughout the day or night. When children cannot or will not clean their teeth, a couple of pieces of xylitol gum will take away any mouth acidity and help them protect their teeth. Medicines that dry the mouth or are sweetened with sugar can aggravate dental problems. Children who take Ritalin will have mouth dryness and often experience a sudden worsening of their teeth and gum conditions. Such problems worsen when children eat or drink acidic foods or beverages, particularly at night. Many young children have dental damage following a bout of sickness, especially if the child has acid reflux or if he or she consumed acidic drinks (like apple juice) during a prolonged period of dehydration or fever. Xylitol offers protection from such drinks or medications. Xylitol made into a liquid drink may be a useful option.

Children with chronic ear infections frequently experience acid reflux, which will damage teeth severely. Use xylitol often to reduce the problem of mouth acidity. Nasal sprays containing xylitol in saline can also help (for example, Xlear nasal spray) and are found in most health food stores and also on the Internet. Xylitol nasal wash may help relieve the symptoms of sinus infections and allergies, too, and it is safe to use for infants and small children.

Preteens and Teens

At age eleven, premolar teeth on the sides of the mouth are coming in, baby teeth will continue to fall out, and the twelve-year molars begin to erupt. This is a critical time to protect teeth. For the first time, permanent teeth are lining up in the mouth, side by side, and touching one other. Cavity-causing bacteria can easily get caught between these new teeth. Flossing may help a little, but may not stop cavities. The best prevention is to make sure the mouth is populated with healthy bacteria. The routine of proper brushing, rinsing with fluoride, and using xylitol becomes the key to dental health for a preteen. This is the time to start your child on the complete program for adults.

A study of teenagers who used a preventive program showed that they could control harmful bacteria in their mouths and reduce the chance of cavities by 80 to 90 percent. The teens simply chewed six to ten pieces of gum sweetened with 100 percent xylitol throughout each day. Protective night and morning rinsing gave complete protection.

Ensuring that newly erupted teeth populate with healthy bacteria protects a teenager's teeth in the same way baby teeth are protected by healthy bacteria when they first erupt. The idea of controlling dental disease by controlling bacteria is new to people, but it is a powerful preventive tool. It is most effective if used at specific times and definitely in the six-month period before tooth eruption.

The late preteen and early teen years are the time when many new permanent teeth take the place of baby teeth. Premolar teeth erupt around ten to fourteen years of age, and second molars come in at the back of the mouth by age fourteen.

Wisdom teeth erupt in the late teen years at the very back of the mouth, usually in places that are difficult to clean. If these teeth are colonized or covered with healthy bacteria, they will not be harmed, provided the mouth is protected from acidity. It is important to emphasize that acidic mouths encourage the growth of harmful bacteria. Teenagers need the xylitol and adult rinsing system protective program to maintain healthy bacteria and protect their new teeth.

Teenagers are prone to acidic mouth conditions for a variety of reasons. Hormonal changes dry the mouth, making it acidic, and at the same time thirsty. Juice drinks, soda, sports drinks, and fruited waters create more acidity that damages teeth directly and also encourages the growth of harmful cavity-forming germs. Sports activity or difficulty closing the mouth because of braces can cause a dry mouth, dehydrated teeth, and reduced natural protection. Fast-food diets can be high in sodium and also create increased thirst. Adolescence is also a time when lack of interest or motivation makes oral hygiene a low priority. Harmful bacteria will grow and flourish in a dirty mouth.

These "perfect storm" conditions foster foul-smelling bacteria. Teenagers concerned about their bad breath may think that chewing gum or eating a breath mint will protect them from the condition, but most gums and mints just mask the odor for a short time and, worse, contain sugar or sorbitol, which feeds harmful germs and helps them multiply. Mints and gum containing sorbitol are often advertised as sugar free, which is confusing. When sorbitol is eaten regularly, harmful plaque bacteria are able to use sorbitol for growth. Alternating sugar and sorbitol may create damaging conditions in the mouth. Closely scrutinize the ingredients of candies and products that are consumed often or eaten before bedtime.

Let your teenager know that xylitol is a great breath freshener. Xylitol also makes teeth shiny and smooth. Teenagers will like the fact that xylitol is all natural and tastes great. Studies show that xylitol and fluoride work in harmony and can strengthen and protect teeth. A teen with bad breath may also like to use the chlorine-dioxide rinse (Closys). When used before brushing and without any added flavoring, this mouth rinse has an immediate effect on bad breath. People have told me that the worst bad breath has disappeared within a week.

Despite the problems associated with the teen years, simple methods can overcome the challenges and give teens the opportunity to reach adulthood with great teeth. Don't fight about toothbrushing: have your teen eat xylitol! When teeth are covered in plaque, poor quality toothbrushing will be of little help anyway. It is more useful to have your child eat xylitol mints and chew xylitol gum and use a good-tasting fluoride rinse to freshen his or her mouth. These products provide protection by removing acids and loosening harmful bacteria from teeth and inactivating them.

Gum disease usually starts during adolescence because of hormonal changes related to puberty that increase risk factors. Prevention is easier than a cure, so young adults need to prevent disease, especially if they have or are about to have braces.

Another important subject for teens is that of bleaching teeth. To summarize the material presented in chapter 10, home-applied bleaching kits and strips can irritate gums. Take great care to avoid touching the gums with the bleaching materials. If bleaching teeth makes your teen more confident and happier, the procedure might be worth considering, but you both need to know that when you bleach teeth, you are removing the protective layer, making the teeth more porous and sensitive, and potentially damaging the gums.

Rinsing with fluoride after bleaching teeth provides a protective layer and encourages the enamel to re-harden, which prevents the teeth from staining. Many fluoride rinses are colored, so you may prefer to use a white toothpaste containing fluoride for this job. Gently brush teeth with a sodium-fluoride-containing toothpaste (Crest original is one) and before spitting or rinsing, swish an ounce (about one tablespoon) of water around your mouth. This technique makes a white fluoride slurry rinse to harden your softened teeth. Be very careful and use fluoride and xylitol as much as possible after bleaching to repair the damage and reduce sensitivity it may have caused.

Braces for Adults and Teens

Braces and orthodontic appliances can make tooth cleaning very difficult. Braces also can prevent lips from closing tightly. Air entering and leaving through the mouth will dry teeth, leaving them unprotected and at increased risk for damage and cavities. Many orthodontists worry about this risk because they have seen the damage that can occur—often in a very short time. But some dentists do not address dental disease and put braces on teeth in an infected mouth where cavities have formed and recently required filling. This is a recipe for disaster. Sometimes parents believe that the orthodontist will be checking the health of their child's teeth during treatment, but not all orthodontists do.

Teeth can be scarred during their time in braces, leaving white marks and softened areas and even cavities. The brackets and wires easily trap harmful bacteria, and in those hidden places, acids produced by the bacteria demineralize the enamel beneath them. A mother recently told me how her thirteen-year-old has been seeing a dentist regularly since she was small. The girl needed a few fillings each year, despite her efforts to limit sugar and brush and floss in the way she had been instructed. The dentist put braces on her teeth to straighten them. When the braces were removed two years later, the girl needed fifteen fillings in her permanent teeth!

The mother feels sad, guilty, and concerned. I am sorry that such a thing occurred, when effective preventive measures before putting in the braces could have avoided the situation. Dental disease is progressive and destructive. Once the disease is in the mouth, it will continue unchecked, constantly causing damage, unless the chemistry of the mouth is changed and the harmful bacteria eliminated.

The easiest and one of the most effective ways to eradicate harmful bacteria is to eat at least 6.5 grams of xylitol every day for six months. Using this "cleansing" program before the braces go onto teeth ensures mouth health before treatment begins. The complete adult routine of mouth rinsing will prepare and strengthen enamel before treatment. If continued during orthodontic treatment, the mouth rinse routine and eating xylitol will prevent bleeding gums, bad breath, and cavities.

I recommend my adult program for anyone with adult teeth, especially anyone with braces or retainers or who has difficulty flossing. This complete system protects and strengthens teeth, and because the taste is good, compliance is great. Whenever mouth conditions are challenging, teeth should be strengthened and protected more than at any other time in life. This preventive program works well for anyone who has braces because it is simple and user friendly. Anyone concerned about maintaining oral health will be happy that the results are cleaner-feeling teeth, fresher breath, and fewer, happier dental visits.

Frequently Asked Questions

Additional questions and answers about preventive dentistry are available at:

www.CleanWhiteTeeth.com

AskDrEllie.blogspot.com

www.Zellies.com

Q: WHAT IS XYLITOL?

A: Xylitol is a naturally occurring sweetener found in the fibers of many fruits and vegetables, including berries, corn husks, oats, and mushrooms. The Finnish name for it is *koivusokeri,* or birch sugar, and it was first produced in Scandinavia from *xylan*, a sugar found in the wood fibers of birch trees.

Q: IS XYLITOL SAFE? WHAT IS A SAFE DOSE?

A: Xylitol is FDA approved and has been safely used by diabetics for more than a hundred years. For dental health, at least six to ten grams (approximately two teaspoons) of xylitol daily are recommended. Xylitol comes from natural sources and has a low glycemic index. Small amounts of xylitol (fifteen grams) are produced naturally in our bodies every day. You can safely eat fifty to a hundred grams a day, but the best advice is to increase the dose slowly.

Q: HOW OFTEN SHOULD I EAT XYLITOL?

A: Every time you use xylitol, in any form or amount, you are protecting and strengthening your teeth. Eating at least six grams of Xylitol in small, divided doses throughout the day will eliminate harmful bacteria in dental plaque in about five weeks. Xylitol moistens a dry mouth and can safely be used to protect your teeth after eating and drinking, day or night.

Q: ARE ALL SUGAR-FREE PRODUCTS GOOD FOR TEETH?

A: Look at the ingredient label. Products containing sorbitol, mannitol, or maltitol may cause gastric problems even at low dosage (these can start with as little as half a teaspoon). Products containing the artificial sweetener sorbitol may actually increase the number of bad bacteria in your mouth. Many diet or sugar-free drinks are very acidic. Low-calorie or diabetic products sweetened with 100 percent xylitol are much better for your health.

Q: ARE THERE OTHER HEALTH BENEFITS TO USING XYLITOL?

A: Studies have shown up to a 40 percent reduction of ear infections in children, as xylitol appears to have beneficial effects on bacteria in the ear tubes that connect with the throat. Some people have experienced relief from the symptoms of acid reflux and heartburn by eating xylitol. If you suffer from allergies or asthma, you may find that a nasal wash containing xylitol can help relieve some of the symptoms. Xylitol is now being incorporated in skin care and cosmetic products.

Q: IS IT POSSIBLE TO REPLACE DAILY TOOTH CLEANING WITH XYLITOL?

A: Xylitol works to make plaque bacteria less sticky and more easily brushed off teeth. Brushing is an excellent way to clean teeth, and appears most important for the health of the gums. In situations where brushing is difficult or impossible, xylitol offers protection for teeth. When toothpaste cannot be tolerated by babies, children, and some adults, use a liquid solution of xylitol to clean the teeth.

Q: CAN XYLITOL CURE BAD BREATH AND WHITEN MY TEETH?

A: An acidic mouth promotes the growth of bacteria that cause bad breath and soften your teeth, allowing them to become worn and stained. Xylitol balances mouth acidity, eliminates acid-producing bacteria, and replaces minerals in teeth, making them stronger and appear brighter.

Q: IS XYLITOL SAFE FOR PETS?

A: A word of caution to pet owners: xylitol is toxic to pets (as are chocolate and raisins). Consumption can lead to serious illness in pets, so take precautions to keep all products that contain xylitol stored safely away from them.

Glossary

anaerobic—existing in the absence of oxygen

biofilm—a resistant layer of bacteria that coats teeth

cariostatic—acting to halt tooth decay

catalyst—an agent that provokes or speeds significant change

cavity—the caving in of a tooth surface following progressive weakening of the surface by acidic attack

cementoenamel junction—the place where tooth enamel joins the root surface of a tooth, and the point where gum tissues meet teeth in a healthy mouth

demineralization—a loss of bodily minerals that weakens the structure

dental caries—a progressive and destructive disease that attacks teeth

dentin—porous, creamy white layer that composes the principal mass of a tooth, within an outer protective layer and encasing live tissue in the center of a tooth

enamel—a mesh of collagen packed with minerals that forms a protective coating over teeth

erosion (tooth)—the act of teeth wearing away following a softening usually caused by acidity

explorer—sharp, pointed instrument that dentists use to check for cavities and tooth decay

fluorosis—mottling of the teeth caused by fluoride as it interferes with enamel formation and results in a speckled or mottled appearance of enamel

gingivitis—a reversible inflammation of the gums, most often seen as bleeding gums

halo effect—the spreading of fluoride from one geographic area to another when food or beverages produced in one place are bought and consumed in another

periodontitis—a more severe progression of gingivitis that occurs when the fibers of tooth attachment become infected and disrupted below the gum line

porous—permeable to liquids

remineralization (tooth)—the rebuilding of minerals into enamel to repair and replace missing minerals and strength

tartar—encrustration of plaque on the teeth

white spot lesions—the first stage of a cavity seen with the naked eye when minerals are lost and the tooth surface weakens and becomes porous

xylitol—a natural sugarless sweetener that has dental and general health properties

Notes

CHAPTER 1

1. R. M. Stephan. "Intra-Oral Hydrogen-Ion Concentration Associated with Dental Caries Activity." *Journal of Dental Research* 23 (1944): 251–66. For diagrams of Stephan graphs, go to www.cleanwhiteteeth.com.

2. J. D. B. Featherstone, "The Science and Practice of Caries Prevention." *Journal of the American Dental Association* 131 (2000): 887–99. See also Featherstone. "Caries Prevention and Reversal Based on the Caries Balance." *Pediatric Dentistry* 28 (2006): 128–32.

3. J. D. B. Featherstone. "The Caries Balance: The Basis for Caries Management by Risk Assessment." *Oral Health and Preventive Dentistry* 2 (2004): 259–64.

4. M. J. Tyas et al. "Minimal Intervention in the Management of Dental Caries—A Review." Federation Dentaire Internationale Commission Project 1–97. *International Dental Journal* 50 (2000): 1–12. Available at www. fdiworldental.org/search/search_asp.asp?txtSearch=minimal+intervention. See also J. White. "Rationale and Treatment Approach in Minimally Invasive Dentistry." *Journal of the American Dental Association* 231 (2000): 12–19.

5. J. White. "Rationale and Treatment Approach in Minimally Inventive Dentistry." *Journal of the American Dental Association* 231 (2000): 12–19. See also C. A. Murdoch-Kinch and M. E. McLean. "Minimally Invasive Dentistry." *Journal of the American Dental Association* (Jan. 2003): 87–95.

6. Tyas et al., "Minimal Intervention."

7. Elliott Moskowitz. Editorial: "Protecting Dentistry's Image." *New York State Dental Journal* (June 2006).

8. "Diagnosis and Management of Dental Caries Throughout Life." NIH Consensus Development Conference, March 2001, Bethesda, MD. *Journal of Dental Education* 65 (2001): 1162.

9. C. Penning et al. "Validity of Probing for Fissure Caries Diagnosis." *Caries Research* 26 (1992): 445–49. See also M. W. Dodds. "Dilemmas in Caries Diagnosis: Applications to Current Practice and Need for Research." *Journal of Dental Education* 57(1993): 433–38.

10. D. A. Young. "New Caries Detection Technologies and Modern Caries Management: Merging the Strategies." *General Dentistry* 50 (2002): 320–31. Available at www.cdafoundation.org/journal/jour0303/stewart.htm.

11. Y. L. and E. H. Verdonschot. "Performance of Diagnostic Systems in Occlusal Caries Detection Compared." *Community Dentistry and Oral Epidemiology* 22 (1994): 187–91. See also N. B. Pitts and P. A. Rimmer. "An In Vivo Comparison of Radiographic and Directly Assessed Clinical Caries Status of Posterior Approximal Surfaces in Primary and Permanent Teeth." *Caries Research* 26 (1992): 146–52.

12. E. A. Kidd, I. Mejare, and B. Nyvad. "Clinical and Radiographic Diagnosis." In O. Ferjerskov and E. A. Kidd, eds. *Dental Caries: The Disease and Its Clinical Management* (Malden, MA: Blackwell, 2003), 111–28.

13. J. C. Hamilton and G. Stookey. "Should a Dental Explorer Be Used to Probe Suspected Carious Lesions?" *Journal of the American Dental Association* 136 (2005): 1526–31.

14. K. R. Ekstrand et al. "Relationship Between External and Histologic Features of Progressive Stages of Caries in the Occlusal Fossa." *Caries Research* 29 (1995): 243–50.

15. P. A. Mileman, H. Mulder, and L. van der Weele. "Factors Influencing the Likelihood of Successful Decisions to Treat Dentin Caries from Bitewing Radiographs." *Community Dentistry and Oral Epidemiology* 20 (1992): 175–80.

16. Department of Protection of the Human Environment. Geneva, Switzerland, a World Health Organization policy paper, "Mercury in Health Care." Available at www.who.int/water_sanitation_health/medicalwaste/mercurypolpaper.pdf. This website describes a 2005 protest at an American Dental Association (ADA) event by a "victim" of mercury poisoning. A poll in 2005 showed that 40 percent of respondents did not know silver fillings were composed of 50 percent mercury. Available at www.madhattersyndrome.com. See also a debate of amalgam issues with a historical overview at www.amalgam.org/#anchor48394.

17. This is the 2002 ADA examination of mercury in dental amalgams. Available at www.ada.org/prof/resources/positions/statements/amalgam 5asp.

18. The Agency for Toxic Substances and Disease Registry describes human health aspects related to mercury. Page 11, which describes the relationship with dental amalgam fillings, is available at www.who.int/ipcs/publications/cicad/en/cicad50.pdf.

19. An ADA overview of dental materials and a comparison chart are available at www.ada.org/prof/resources/topics/materials/index.asp.

20. L. Trost, M. Scarlett, S. Abrams. "Focus on Dental Caries Management: The Remineralization Challenge," part 2. *Woman Dentist Journal* (Jan. 2004): 24–32.

21. Main home page for the Inspektor Dental Light, used to show weakened areas of teeth. Available at www.inspektor.nl/dental/main.htm.

22. Ibid. See also D. A. Young. "New Caries Detection Technologies and Modern Caries Management: Merging the Strategies." *General Dentistry* 50 (2002): 320–31.

23. S. Abrams and M. Scarlett. "Focus on Dental Caries Management," part 1. *Woman Dentist Journal* (Dec. 2003): 8–14. See also S. Tranaeus et al. "In Vivo Repeatability and Reproduceability of the Quantitative Light-Induced Fluorescence Method." *Caries Research* 36 (2002): 3–9.

24. J. D. B. Featherstone. "The Science and Practice of Caries Prevention." *Journal of the American Dental Association* 131 (2000): 887–99.

25. One website of a mouth fitness dentist is available at www.fitmouth. com.

26. M. H. Anderson, D. J. Bales, and K. A. Omnell. "Modern Management of Dental Caries: The Cutting Edge Is Not the Dental Burr." *Journal of the American Dental Association* 124 (1993): 37–44.

CHAPTER 2

1. G. Montes. "Children's Oral Health: Comparing Rochester Area PACE Data to the National Survey of Children's Health 2003." (Rochester, NY: Children's Institute, Inc., 2006).

2. Centers for Disease Control and Prevention's National Center for Health Statistics Report. Available at www.cdc.gov/nchs/fastats/dental.htm.

3. MetLife Oral Health Insights Study conducted by a market research firm during the third quarter of 2006 among nationally representative sample of 1,200 adults across the United States with ages between 18 and 64. Available at www.webdentistry.com/News-article-sid-2982-theme-Printer. html.

4. A report of the 51st Surgeon General on Oral Health in America. 2000. Available at www.surgeongeneral.gov/library/oralhealth.

5. Richard H. Carmona, MD, MPH, FACS. Surgeon General, U.S. Department of Health and Human Services. A National Oral Health Call to Action. 2003. NIH Publication No. 03-5303. Available at www.surgeongeneral.gov/news/speeches/oralhealth042903.htm.

6. The CDC's Oral Health Resource Library fact sheet explaining the association between the American Association for Dental Research (AADR) and the Health and Human Resources agencies (HHR) with alliances to work on the project "Healthy People 2010—Oral Health Objectives." Available at www.cdc.gov/OralHealth/factsheets/hp2010.htm.

7. J. D. Shenkin et al. "Soft Drink Consumption and Caries Risk in Children and Adolescents." *General Dentistry* 51 (2003): 30–36. See also C. J. Hase and D. Birkhed. "Salivary Glucose Clearance, Dry Mouth and pH Changes in Dental Plaque in Man." *Archives of Oral Biology* 33 (1988): 875–80; and E. H. Roos and K. J. Donly. "In Vivo Dental Plaque pH Variation with Regular and Diet Soft Drinks." *Pediatric Dentistry* 24 (2002): 350–53. Available at www.aapd.org/upload/articles-old/donly7-02.pdf.

8. K. R. Kongara and E. E. Soffer. "Saliva and Esophageal Protection." *American Journal of Gastroenterology* 94 (1999): 1446–52.

CHAPTER 3

1. P. W. Caufield, G. R. Cutter, and A. P. Dasanayake. "Initial Acquisition of Mutans Streptococci by Infants: Evidence for a Discrete Window of Infectivity." *Journal of Dental Research* 72 (1993): 37–45.

2. R. E. Stewart and K. J. Hale. "The Paradigm Shift in the Etiology, Prevention, and Management of Dental Caries: Its Effect on the Practice of Clinical Dentistry." *Journal of the California Dental Association* 31 (2003): 247–52.

3. R. J. Berkowitz. "Acquisition and Transmission of Mutans Streptococci." *Journal of the California Dental Association* 31 (2003): 135–38.

4. Y. Li et al. "Mode of Delivery and Other Maternal Factors Influence the Acquisition of Streptococcus Mutans in Infants." *Journal of Dental Research* 84 (2005): 806–11.

5. W. J. Loesche. "Role of Streptococcus Mutans in Human Dental Decay." *FEMS Microbiology Reviews* 50 (1986): 353–80.

6. R. J. Berkowitz, J. Turner, and P. Green. "Maternal Salivary Levels of Streptococcus Mutans: The Primary Oral Infection in Infants." *Archives of Oral Biology* 26 (1981): 147–49.

7. B. Kohler, D. Bratthall, and B. Krasse. "Preventive Measures in Mothers Influence the Establishment of the Bacterium Streptococcus Mutans in Their Infants." *Archives of Oral Biology* 28 (1983): 225–31.

8. A. K. Wan et al. "Association of Streptococcus Mutans Infection and Oral Developmental Nodules in Pre-dentate Infants." *Journal of Dental Research* 80 (2001): 1945–48. See also S. Alaluusua and O.V. Renkonen. "Streptococcus Mutans Establishment and Dental Caries Experience in Children from 2 to 4 Years Old." *Scandinavian Journal of Dental Research* 91 (1982): 453–57.

9. B. Kohler, I. Andreen, and B. Jonsson. "The Effect of Caries-Preventive Measures in Mothers on Dental Caries and the Oral Presence of the Bacteria Streptococcus Mutans and Lactobacilli in Their Children." *Archives of Oral Biology* 29 (1984): 879–83.

10. P. Isokangas et al. "Occurrence of Dental Decay in Children after Maternal Consumption of Xylitol Chewing Gum, A Follow-up from 0–5 Years of Age." *Journal of Dental Research* 79 (2000): 1885–89. See also E. Soderling et al. "Influence of Maternal Xylitol Consumption on Acquisition of Mutans Streptococci by Infants." *Journal of Dental Research* 79 (2000): 882–87.

11. New York State Department of Health. "Oral Health Care during Pregnancy and Early Childhood. Practice Guidelines." August 2006. Available at www.cda.org/library/pdfs/pregnancy_care.pdf.

12. R. O. Mattos-Graner et al. "Genotypic Diversity of Mutans Streptococci in Brazilian Nursery Children Suggests Horizontal Transmission." *Journal of Clinical Microbiology* 39 (2001): 13–18.

CHAPTER 4

1. W. J. Loesche et al. "Association of Streptococcus Mutans with Human Dental Decay." *Infectious Immunology* 11 (1975): 1252–60.

2. J. J. de Soet, B. Nyvad, and M. Kilian. "Strain-Related Acid Production by Oral Streptococci." *Caries Research* 34 (2000): 486–90.

3. R. M. Stephan. "Changes in Hydrogen-Ion Concentration on Tooth Surfaces and in Carious Lesions." *Journal of the American Dental Association* 27 (1940): 718–23.

4. B. E. Gustafsson et al. "The Vipeholm Dental Caries Study." *Acta Odontologica Scandinavia* 11 (1954): 232–364.

5. R. M. Stephan. "Intra-Oral Hydrogen-Ion Concentration Associated with Dental Caries Activity." *Journal of Dental Research* 23 (1944): 251–66.

6. J. D. B. Featherstone. "The Science and Practice of Caries Prevention." *Journal of the American Dental Association* 131 (2000): 887–99. Available at www.ucsf.edu/cmb/featherstone.htm.

7. Anderson et al., ibid. See also K. J. Anusavice. "Treatment Regimens in Preventive and Restorative Dentistry." *Journal of the American Dental Association* 126 (1995): 727–43.

8. K. J. Anusavice. "Efficacy of Nonsurgical Management of the Initial Caries Lesion." *Journal of Dental Education* 61 (1997): 895–905.

9. J. M. ten Cate, J. J. M. Damen, and M. J. Buijs. "Inhibition of Dentin Demineralization by Fluoride in Vitro." *Caries Research* 32 (1998): 141–47. See also M. J. Larsen, E. I. F. Pearce, and S. J. Jensen. "Notes on the Dissolution of Human Dental Enamel in Dilute Acid Solutions at High Solid/ Solution Ratio." *Caries Research* 27 (1993): 87–95; and J. D. B. Featherstone. "Prevention and Reversal of Dental Caries: Role of Low-Level Fluoride." *Community Dentistry and Oral Epidemiology* 27 (1999): 31–40.

10. J. D. B. Featherstone et al. "A Randomized Clinical Trial of Caries Management by Risk Assessment." *Caries Research* 39 (2005): 295.

CHAPTER 5

1. L. K. Banan and A. M. Hedge. "Plaque and Salivary pH Changes after Consumption of Fresh Fruit Juices." *Journal of Clinical Pediatric Dentistry* 30 (2005): 9–13.

2. pH testing paper is available for purchase at www.zellies.com.

3. J. Tenovuo. "Salivary Parameters of Relevance for Assessing Caries Activity in Individuals and Populations." *Community Dentistry and Oral Epidemiology* 25 (1997): 82–86.

4. B. Krasse. "Biological Factors as Indicators of Future Caries." *International Dental Journal* 38 (1988): 219–25.

5. A. Bardow, B. Nyvad, and B. Nauntofte. "Relationships between Medication Intake, Complaints of Dry Mouth, Salivary Rate and Composition, and the Rate of Tooth Demineralization in Situ." *Archives of Oral Biology* 46 (2001): 413–23.

6. J. D. B. Featherstone. "The Caries Balance: The Basis for Caries Management by Risk Assessment." *Oral Health and Preventive Dentistry* 2 (2004): 259–64.

7. J. M. Tanzer. "Salivary and Plaque Microbiological Tests and the Management of Dental Caries." *Journal of Dental Education* 61 (1997): 866–75. See also A. Hall and J. M. Girkin. "A Review of Potential New Diagnostic Modalities for Caries Lesions." *Journal of Dental Research* 83 (2004): 89–94.

CHAPTER 6

1. W. D. Miller. *The Micro-Organisms of the Human Mouth: The Local and General Diseases Which Are Caused by Them.* (Philadelphia: S.S. White, 1890; republished Basel: S. Karger, 1973).

2. "Symposium on the Prevention of Oral Disease in Children and Adolescents." Conference Papers. *Pediatric Dentistry* 28 (2006): 95–191.

3. M. H. Anderson and W. Shi. "A Probiotic Approach to Caries Management." *Pediatric Dentistry* 28 (2006): 151–53.

4. F. R. von der Fehr, H. Loe, and E. Theilade. "Experimental Caries in Man." *Caries Research* 4 (1970): 131–48.

5. P. Axelsson and J. Lindhe. "The Effect of a Preventive Programme on Dental Plaque, Gingivitis and Caries in School Children: Results after One and Two Years." *Journal of Clinical Periodontology* 1 (1974): 126–38.

6. H. J. Keene and I. L. Shklair. "Relationship of Streptococcus Mutans Carrier Status to the Development of Carious Lesions in Initially Caries-Free Recruits." *Journal of Dental Research* 53 (1974): 1295.

7. P. D. Marsh and D. J. Bradshaw. "Microbial Community Aspects of Dental Plaque." In H. N. Newman and M. Wilson, eds. *Dental Plaque Revisited: Oral Biofilms in Health and Disease* (Cardiff: BioLine, 1999), 237–53.

8. P. D. Marsh. "Microbial Ecology of Dental Plaque and Its Significance in Health and Disease." *Advances in Dental Research* 8 (1994): 263–71.

CHAPTER 7

1. Richard H. Carmona, MD, MPH, FACS. "Surgeon General, U.S. Department of Health and Human Services. A National Oral Health Call to Action." NIH Publication No. 03-5303, 2003. Available at www.surgeongeneral.gov/news/speeches/oralhealth042903.htm.

2. American Academy of Periodontology reference sites for links between gum condition and heart disease, diabetes, pregnancy outcome, and women's health:
www.perio.org/consumer/mbc.heart.htm
www.perio.org/consumer/type2-diabetes.htm
www.perio.org/consumer/pregnancy.htm#2
www.perio.org/consumer/women_resources.htm#news.

3. American Academy for Cancer Research Fifth Annual International Conference on Frontiers in Cancer Prevention Research. Boston. "How Diet, Obesity and Even Gum Disease May Affect Immune System and Cancer" (Nov. 2006).

4. M. K. Jeffcoat, J. C. Hauth, and N. C. Geurs. "Periodontal Disease and Pre-term Birth: Results of a Pilot Intervention Study." *Journal of Periodontology* 74 (2003): 1214–18.

5. B. S. Michalowicz et al. "Treatment of Periodontal Disease and the Risk of Preterm Birth." *New England Journal of Medicine* 355 (2006): 1885–94. Available at www.content.nejm.org/cgi/content/full/355/18/1885?ijkey=oq. onAGFYLSrw&keytype=ref&siteid=nejm.

6. G. H. Hildebrandt and B. S. Sparks. "Maintaining Mutans Streptococci Suppression with Xylitol Chewing Gum." *Journal of the American Dental Association* 131 (2000): 909–16.

7. J. A. Ship. "Diabetes and Oral Health: An Overview." *Journal of the American Dental Association* 134 (2003): 4–10. See also G. W. Taylor. "The Effects of Periodontal Treatment on Diabetes." *Journal of the American Dental Association* 124 (2003): 41–48.

CHAPTER 8

1. Val Valerian. A Chronology of Fluoridation. Available at www.curezone.com/dental/fluoride.html.

2. D. G. Pendrys and R.V. Katz. "Risk for Enamel Fluorosis Associated with Fluoride Supplementation, Infant Formula and Fluoride Dentifrice Use." *American Journal Epidemiology* 130 (1989): 1199–1208. See also O. Fejerskov, J. Ekstrand, and B. A. Burt. *Fluoride in Dentistry*, 2d ed. (Copenhagen: Munksgaard, 1996).

3. C. Bryson. *The Fluoride Deception* (New York: Seven Stories Press, 2004).

4. 2000 Review of Toxicological Literature for Aluminum Compounds for the National Institute of Environmental Health Sciences. Available at

www.ntp.niehs.nih.gov/ntp/htdocs/Chem_Background/ExSumPdf/Aluminum.pdf.

5. O. Fejerskov, F. Manji, and V. Baelum. "The Nature and Mechanisms of Dental Fluorosis in Man." *Journal Dental Research* 69 (1990): 692–700.

6. Links to information about water filtration to remove fluoride: www.friendsofwater.com/Water_Purifiers.html www.equinox-products.com/FluorideMaster.htm.

7. D. G. Pendrys, R.V. Katz, and D. R. Morse. "Risk Factors for Enamel Fluorosis in a Fluoridated Population." *American Journal of Epidemiology* 140 (1994): 461–71.

8. S. M. Adair. "Evidence-Based Use of Fluoride in Contemporary Pediatric Dental Practice." *Pediatric Dentistry* 28 (2006): 133–42. See also "Fluoride Recommendations Work Group: Recommendations for Using Fluoride to Prevent and Control Dental Caries in the United States" (Government Printing Office, Aug. 2001).

9. S. M. Levy et al. "Infants' Fluoride Intake from Drinking Water Alone, and from Water Added to Formula, Beverages and Food." *Journal of Dental Research* 74 (1995): 1399–1407. See also S. Van Winkle et al. "Water and Formula Fluoride Concentrations: Significance for Infants Fed Formula." *Pediatric Dentistry* 17 (1995): 305–10.

10. H. M. van Rijkom, G. J. Truin, and M. A. van Hof. "Caries-Inhibiting Effect of Professional Fluoride Gel Application in Low-Caries Children Initially Aged 4.5–6.5 Years." *Caries Research* 38 (2004): 115–23.

11. Summary of the clinical recommendations from the Council on Scientific Affairs. Available at www.ada.org/prof/resources/pubs/jada/reports/report fluoride_exec.pdf.

CHAPTER 9

1. I. G. Chestnutt et al. "The Prevalence and Effectiveness of Fissure Sealants in Scottish Adolescents." *British Dental Journal* 77 (1994): 125–29.

2. J. B. Dennison, L. H. Straffon, and R. C. Smith. "Effectiveness of Sealant Treatment over Five Years in an Insured Population." *Journal of the American Dental Association* 131 (2000): 597–605.

3. R. J. Feigal. "Sealant and Preventive Restorations: Review of Effectiveness and Clinical Changes for Improvement." *Pediatric Dentistry* 20 (1998): 85–92.

4. P. Alanen. M. I. Holsti, and K. Pienihakkinen. "Sealants and Xylitol Chewing Gum Are Equal in Caries Prevention." *Acta Odontologica Scandinavia* 58 (2000): 279–84.

CHAPTER 10

1. Oral Health Policy: Dental Bleaching for Child and Adolescent Patients. Council on Clinical Affairs. Pediatric Dentistry. Reference Manual.

2. J. D. Shulman et al. "Perceptions of Desirable Tooth Color among Parents, Dentists, and Children." *Journal of the American Dental Association* 135 (2004): 599.

3. K. J. Donly et al. "Tooth Whitening in Children." *Compendium of Continuing Education in Dentistry* 23 (2002): 22–28.

4. P. Moreira de Frietas et al. "Monitoring of Demineralized Dentin Micro-Hardness throughout and after Bleaching." *American Journal of Dentistry* 17 (2004): 346.

5. H. Albers. "Lightening Natural Teeth." *ADEPT Report* 2 (1991): 1–24.

6. S. C. Cohen and C. Chase. "Human Pulpal Response to Bleaching Procedures on Vital Teeth." *Journal of Endodontics* 5 (1979): 134–38.

7. K. B. Frazier and V. B. Haywood. "Teaching Night-Guard Bleaching and Other Tooth Whitening Procedures in North American Dental Schools." *Journal of Dental Education* 64 (2000): 357–64.

8. G. Gambarini et al. "Efficacy and Safety Assessment of a New Liquid Tooth Whitening Gel Containing 5.9 Percent Hydrogen Peroxide." *American Journal of Dentistry* 17 (2004): 78.

9. L.V. Powell and D. J. Bales. "Tooth Bleaching: Its Effect on Oral Tissues." *Journal of the American Dental Association* 122 (1991): 50–54.

10. T. P. Croll. "Tooth Bleaching for Children and Teens: A Protocol and Examples." *Quintessence International* 25 (1994): 811–17.

11. A. Ito et al. "Correlation between Induction of Duodenal Tumor by Hydrogen Peroxide and Catalase Activity in Mice." *Gann* 75 (1982): 17–21.

12. "Data Linking Hydrogen Peroxide and Cancerous Lesions Is Withdrawn." *New York State Dental Journal* 65 (1999): 37.

13. M. G. D. Kelleher and F. J. C. Roe. "The Safety in Use of 10 Percent Carbamide Peroxide (Opalescence) for Bleaching Teeth under the Supervision of a Dentist." *British Dental Journal* (1999): 187. Available at www.nature.com/bdj/journal/v187/n4/full/4800237a.html.

14. S. L. Zouain-Ferreira et al. "Radiation Induced–Like Effects of Four Home Bleaching Agents Used for Tooth Whitening Effect on Bacterial Cultures with Different Capabilities of Reducing Deoxyribonucleic Acid (DNA) Damage." *Cellular and Molecular Biology* 48 (2002): 521–24.

15. The Supplemental Guidance for Assessing Cancer Susceptibility Review Panel of the EPA Science Advisory Board. Review of the EPA's Draft Supplemental Guidance for Assessing Cancer Susceptibility from Early Life

Exposure to Carcinogens. Washington, DC: EPA, March 2004. Publication (EPA-SAB) No. 04-003.

16. J. E. Dahl and U. Pallesen. "Tooth Bleaching—A Critical Review of the Biological Aspects." *Critical Reviews in Oral Biology and Medicine* 14 (2003): 292–304.

17. K. J. Donly et al. "Effectiveness and Safety of Tooth Bleaching in Teen-agers." *Pediatric Dentistry* 27 (2005): 298–302.

18. N. S. Seale, J. E. McIntosh, and A. N. Taylor. "Pulpal Reaction to Bleaching of Teeth in Dogs." *Journal of Dental Research* 80 (1981): 948–53.

19. N. S. Seale, J. E. McIntosh, and A. N. Taylor. "Pulpal Response of Bleaching of Teeth in Dogs." *Pediatric* Dentistry 7 (1985): 209–14.

20. T. W. Hummert et al. "Mercury in Solution Following Exposure of Various Amalgams to Carbamide Peroxides." *American Journal of Dentistry* 6 (1993): 305–9. See also I. Rotstein, C. Mor, and J. R. Arwac. "Changes in Surface Levels of Mercury, Silver, Tin and Copper of Dental Amalgam Treated with Carbamide Peroxide and Hydrogen Peroxide in Vitro." *Oral Surgery, Oral Medicine, Oral Pathology, Oral Radiology and Endodontology* 83 (1997): 506–9.

CHAPTER 11

1. S. D. Hogg and A. J. Rugg-Gunn. "Can the Oral Flora Adapt to Sorbitol?" *Journal of Dentistry* 19 (1991): 263–71. See also E. Soderling et al. "Effect of Sorbitol, Xylitol and Xylitol/Sorbitol Chewing Gums on Dental Plaque." *Caries Research* 23 (1989): 378–84.

2. M. A. Gales and T. M. Nguyen. "Sorbitol Compared with Xylitol in the Prevention of Dental Caries." *Annals of Pharmacotherapy* 34 (2000): 98–100.

3. P. Milgrom et al. "Mutans Streptococci Dose Response to Xylitol Chewing Gum." *Journal of Dental Research* 85 (2006): 177–81.

4. E. H. Roos and K. J. Donly. "In Vivo Dental Plaque pH Variation with Regular and Diet Soft Drinks." *Pediatric Dentistry* 24 (2002): 350–53. Available at www.aapd.org/upload/articles-old/donly7-02.pdf.

5. R. Hartmink et al. "Degradation and Fermentation of Fructooligosaccharides by Oral Streptococci." *Journal of Applied Bacteriology* 79 (1995): 551–57. See also P. G. Roberts and M. L. Hayes. "Effects of 2-Deoxy-D-Glucose and Other Sugar Analogues on Acid Production from Sugars by Human Dental Plaque Bacteria." *Scandinavian Journal of Dental Research* 88 (1980): 201–9.

6. Dr. Joseph Mercola with Dr. Kendra Degen Pearsall. *Sweet Deception: Why Splenda, Nutrasweet and the FDA May Be Hazardous to Your Health* (Nashville, TN: Nelson Books, 2006).

7. M. A. Gales and T. M. Nguyen. "Sorbitol Compared with Xylitol in the Prevention of Dental Caries." *Annals of Pharmacotherapy* 34 (2000): 98–100.

8. S. D. Hogg and A. J. Rugg-Gunn. "Can the Oral Flora Adapt to Sorbitol?" *Journal of Dentistry* 19 (1991): 263–71.

9. P. L. Holgerson et al. "Dental Plaque Formation and Salivary Mutans Streptococci in Schoolchildren after Use of Xylitol-Containing Chewing Gum." *International Journal of Pediatric Dentistry* 17 (2007): 79–85.

10. D. Brownstein. *Salt: Your Way to Health* (West Bloomfield Township, MI: Medical Alternatives Press, 2006).

11. Mineral Waters of the World is a website with alphabetic listings, consumer ratings, and the ability to search for mineral water pH measurements. This information is available at www.mineralwaters.org.

12. One website for information about water testing is www.aquamd.com/diagnostic.

13. Baby care tooth wipes with xylitol are available for purchase from www.spiffies.com.

14. M. E. Thompson, J. G. Dever, and E. I. F. Pearce. "Intra-Oral Testing of Flavoured Sweetened Milk." *New Zealand Dental Journal* 80 (1984): 44–46.

15. W. H. Bowen et al. "Influence of Milk, Lactose-Reduced Milk and Lactose on Caries in Desalivated Rats." *Caries Research* 25 (1991): 283–86.

16. P. J. Moynihan, S. Ferrier, and G. N. Jenkins. "The Cariostatic Potential of Cheese: Cooked Cheese-Containing Meals Increase Plaque Calcium Concentration." *British Dental Journal* 187 (1999): 664–67.

17. I. Gedalia et al. "Dental Caries Protection with Hard Cheese Consumption." *American Journal of Dentistry* 7 (1994): 331–32.

18. B. E. Gustafsson et al. "The Vipeholm Dental Caries Study: The Effect of Different Levels of Carbohydrate Intake on Caries Activity in 436 Individuals Observed for Five Years." *Acta Odontologica Scandinavia* 11 (1954): 232–64.

19. E. J. Gravenmade and G. N. Jenkins. "Isolation, Purification and Some Properties of a Potential Cariostatic Factor in Cocoa That Lowers Enamel Solubility." *Caries Research* 30 (1986): 433–36.

20. D. S. Magrill. "The Reduction of the Solubility of Hydroxyapatite in Acid by Absorption of Phytate from Solution." *Archives of Oral Biology* 18 (1973): 591–600.

21. S. Rosen et al. "Anti-Cariogenic Effects of Tea in Rats." *Journal of Dental Research* 63 (1984): 658–60.

22. M. Daglia et al. "Anti Adhesive Effect of Green and Roasted Coffee on Streptococcus Mutans' Adhesive Properties on Saliva-Coated Hydroxyapatite Beads." *Journal of Agricultural and Food Chemistry* 50 (2002): 1225–29.

23. H. Koo et al. "Influence of Cranberry Juice on Glucan-Mediated Processes Involved in Streptococcus Mutans Biofilm Development." *Caries Research* 40 (2006): 20–27.

24. H. Koo et al. "Effect of a Mouthrinse Containing Selected Propolis on 3-Day Dental Plaque Accumulation and Polysaccharide Formation." *Caries Research* 36 (2002): 445–48.

25. A. P. Dasanayake and P. W. Caufield. "Prevalence of Dental Caries in Sri Lankan Aboriginal Veddha Children." *International Dental Journal* 52 (2002): 438–44. See also P. C. Molan. "The Potential of Honey to Promote Oral Wellness." *General Dentistry* 49 (2001): 583–89.

26. Natural Products. *Bee Honey: The Composition of Honey.* Available at www.naturalproducts.almaleka.com/bproducts/honey /h2.htm.

CHAPTER 12

1. M. Lam et al. "Children's Acceptance of Xylitol-Based Foods." *Community Dentistry and Oral Epidemiology* 28 (2000): 218–24.

2. K. K. Makinen et al. "Stabilization of Rampant Caries: Polyol Gums and Arrest of Dentine Caries in Two Long-Term Cohort Studies in Young Subjects." *International Dental Journal* 45 (1995b): 93–107.

3. P. Alanen, R. Isokangas, and K. Gutmann. "Xylitol Candies in Caries Prevention: Results of a Field Study in Estonian Children." *Community Dentistry and Oral Epidemiology* 28 (2000): 218–24.

4. P. Milgrom et al. "Mutans Streptococci Dose Response to Xylitol Chewing Gum." *Journal of Dental Research* 85 (2006): 177–81.

5. L. Trahan. "Xylitol: A Review of Its Action on Mutans Streptococci and Dental Plaque—Its Clinical Significance." *International Dental Journal* 45 (1995): 77–92. See also P. J. Isokangas et al. "Dental Daries and Mutans

Streptococci in the Proximal Areas of Molars Affected by the Habitual Use of Xylitol Chewing Gum." *Caries Research* 25 (1991): 444–48.

6. A. J. Rugg-Gunn. *Nutrition, Diet and Oral Health* (Oxford: Oxford University Press, 1993).

7. J. O. Klein. "What's New in the Diagnosis and Management of Otitis Media?" *Pediatric Annals* (2002): 777–79. See also T. Kontiokari, M. Niemel, and M. Uhari. "Effect of Xylitol on the Resolution of Middle Ear Effusion in Acute Otitis Media." *Pediatric Research* 45 (1999): 165.

8. Nasal Xylitol. How xylitol can stop the source of sinus, ear infections, allergies and asthma. Available at www.Nasal-Xylitol.com.

9. P. J. Isokangas et al. "Occurrence of Dental Decay in Children after Maternal Consumption of Xylitol Chewing Gum: A Follow-Up from 0–5 Years of Age." *Journal of Dental Research* 79 (2000): 1885–89.

10. R. H. Manning, W. M. Edgar, and E. A. Agamanyi. "Effects of Chewing Gums Sweetened with Sorbitol or a Sorbitol/Xylitol Mixture on the Remineralization of Human Enamel Lesions in Situ." *Caries Research* 26 (1992): 194–209. See also K. Wennerholm et al. "Effect of Xylitol and Sorbitol in Chewing Gums on Mutans Streptococci Plaque pH and Mineral Loss of Enamel." *Caries Research* 28 (1994): 48–54; and K. A. Ly, P. Milgrom, and M. Rothen. "Xylitol, Sweeteners, and Dental Caries." *Pediatric Dentistry* 28 (2006): 154–63.

11. E. Honkala et al. "Field Trial on Caries Prevention with Xylitol Candies among Disabled School Students." *Caries Research* 40 (2006): 508–13.

12. O. Aguirre-Zero, D. T. Zero, and H. M. Proskin. "Effect of Chewing Xylitol Chewing Gum on Salivary Flow Rate and the Acidogenic Potential of Dental Plaque." *Caries Research* 27 (1993): 55–59.

13. Wikipedia provides a description of xylitol and explains its extraction and medical properties. Available at www.en.wikipedia.org/wiki/Xylitol.

14. Information about the army's "Look for Xylitol First" program is available at www.xylitolinfo.com/cms/connect/xylitol/news/news.htm.

15. C. Hayes. "The Effect of Non-Cariogenic Sweeteners on the Prevention of Dental Caries: A Review of the Evidence." *Journal of Dental Education* 65 (2001): 1106–09.

16. H. K. Akerblom et al. "The Tolerance of Increasing Amounts of Dietary Xylitol in Children." *International Journal for Vitamin and Nutrition Research* 22 (1982): 53–66.

17. H. Forster, R. Quadbeck, and U. Gottstein. "Metabolic Tolerance to High Doses of Oral Xylitol in Human Volunteers Not Previously Adapted to Xylitol." *International Journal for Vitamin and Nutrition Research* 22 (1982): 67–88.

18. J. L. Sintes et al. "Enhanced Anti-Caries Efficacy of a 0.243 Percent Sodium Fluoride/10 Percent Xylitol/Silica Dentifrice: 3 Year Clinical Results." *American Journal of Dentistry* 8 (1995): 231–35. See also K. K. Makinen et al. "Biochemical, Microbiologic and Clinical Comparisons between Two Dentifrices That Contain Different Mixtures of Sugar Alcohols." *Journal of the American Dental Association* 111 (1985): 745–51.

CHAPTER 13

1. J. D. B. Featherstone. "Caries Prevention and Reversal Based on the Caries Balance." *Pediatric Dentistry* 28 (2006): 128–32.

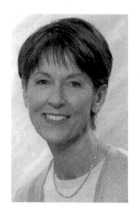

About the Author

Dr. Ellie Phillips has practiced dentistry with a focus on prevention of disease for thirty-five years, treating patients from all walks of life including geriatrics, special-needs children, and the developmentally disabled.

Dr. Ellie is a member of the American Dental Association, the New York State Dental Association, and the American Academy of Pediatric Dentists, and is a founding member and board memeber of the American Academy for Oral Systemic Health. She is a graduate of Eastman Dental Center, Rochester, New York, with qualifications in pediatric and general dentistry. She is an honorary member of the Eastman Academy, University of London, England. In the United States Dr. Ellie was the pediatric outpatient clinic director at the

Eastman Dental Center and a member of faculty at the University of Rochester. She contributed to building a university multidisciplinary private practice dental team and provided care in assisted-living facilities and centers for the developmentally disabled in Rochester.

When Dr. Ellie was in private practice, she particularly enjoyed being able to remove the concerns of the fearful and the phobic.

Says Dr. Ellie: "This system of care has allowed me to keep my own fillings in perfect condition for more than forty years. During this time I have never had a new cavity, filling, or other dental treatment, nor have I experienced sensitivity. I have had only one dental cleaning in the past twenty years. Without following traditional methods of dental care, my teeth have remained healthy, shiny, and cavity free.

"I encourage anyone who is searching for dental health to try this system; clean your toothbrush, store it safely, and get started today."

Index

A
acid-loving bacteria, 42, 59, 73
acidity and tooth damage, 55
acidity,
    avoidance, 60
    caused by, 60–61
    damages, combined with mouth
        dryness, 61
    dental problems, risk for, 61
    source of, 61
alkaline balance, 59–60
Alzheimer's disease, 91
ameloblasts,
    poisoned by, 101
American Dental Association (ADA)
        claims, 12
anaerobic plaque bacteria, 70
ankylosis, 117
atraumatic restorative treatment, 7

B
bacteria,
    inheritance of, 34
    kind of, 33
    saliva-sharing activities, avoid, 35
    transfer, 32
bacterial endocarditis, 80–81
bisphenol, 108
bleaching,
    children's teeth, 121–123
    hydrogen peroxide, released from, 123
    laser, with, 125
    last option, 123
    negative effects of, 117–118, *see also*
        gum recession
    pulp, hemorrhaging and inflammation
        in, 123
    questions to ask before, 125
    silver fillings, affect, 124
braces for adults and teens, 198–199
breast milk, 190–191
burs, 109

C
cancer risk, 120
    bleaching, harmful effect of, 121
    hydrogen peroxide, potential of, 120
carbamide peroxide, problem with, 119
caries and cavities,
    sugar and bacteria, interaction, 41

cementoenamel junction, 76
children's saliva, 62–63
children, mouth care system for , 187
chlorine-dioxide rinse, 168
Closys, 78, 168, 182, 197
cosmetic dental makeovers, 114
    negative study results, 115

D
demineralization, meaning of, 48
dental attitudes, 3
dental caries, 43–44, 156
    bacteria, sugars and starches supply,
        44
    perfect storm conditions, 44
dental cleaning, 71–74
dental disease,
    bacteria, caused by, see bacteria
    dry mouth, 165
    factors, 165
    mouth acidity, 165
    risk for, 164
dental health and general health, 79–80
dental problems,
    dry mouth, 50
    Listerine, use of, 50
dental problems, risk factor, 27
dental training, 5
dentin, 115–117
dentistry,
    history of, 19
    new techniques in, see new techniques
        in dentistry
    new type of, 6
dentists,
    prevention, 4
    evaluators and fitness trainers, 16
    frustration, 29
Dr. Ellie's Dental Care System, 165
    athletes, 184–185
    brush, choosing, 169–171
    diabetics, 185–186
    fluoride rinse, 175
    men, help, 180–181
    pregnant women, helps, 177–180

process, 167
rinse, ingredients in, 174
seniors and those with special needs,
    helps, 182–184
step 1, cleaning prerinse, 167–168
step 2, toothbrushing, 168
step 3, rinse after brushing, 173
toothpaste, choosing, 172–173
women, helps, 176–177
dry adolescent mouth, 50–52

E
Eastman Dental Center, 24–25
enamel,
    acidic mouth liquid, role of, 46
    bleaching, effect of, 115
    composition, 46, see also minerals
    fluoride, role of, 47
    protection, 45
explorer, meaning of, 9
    cavity finding, unreliable technique
        for, 9

F
filling,
    material, health impact, 8
    time of, 10–11
    type of, 12
flossing, usefulness of, 28
fluoride,
    absorption of minerals, increase, 100
    aluminum, affinity for, 91–93
    ameloblasts, see ameloblasts
    children's teeth, 100
    high-concentration product, avoid, 98
    history of, 88–90
    maturation, increased, 101
    misconceptions, 93–95
    mouth rinse, 97–100
    pros and cons of, 90–91
    sources of, 95–96
    treatments, 104
    varnish, 105–106, 153, 193
    weak and strong, 99
    weak fluoride, catalyst, 99

xylitol, combined with, 103
fluorosis, 89, 96, 101–102
focus of infection theory, 79
food for teeth,
    balance, achieving, 130
    cariostatic food, 139
    cheese and chocolate, 140–141
    citric acid, 136–137
    coconut milk, 143
    cow's milk, 139–140
    diet and energy drinks, 138
    honey, cause cavity, 143
    intense sweeteners, 142
    oligosaccharides, 133
    plant fibers and leaves, 141
    propolis, 142
    spiffies, 139, 183, 189
    sugar substitutes, 130–131
    sugar-free foods, damage, 132–134
    water, acidity, alkalinity measurement
        of, 135
    xylitol *versus* sorbitol, 131–132
    xylitol, protection with, 138–139

G
germs protect, 68
gingivitis, 75–78
    Listerine, role of, 174
gold, porcelain filling, 14
gum disease,
    kinds of, 75
    preterm births, 81
    prevention, 82–83, *see also* xylitol
gum recession, 119–120

H
halo effect, 96
healthy bones and teeth, maintenance, 46
healthy plaque, 69–71
home-treatment methods, 16–17
hydroxyl-free radical, 119

I
incomplete lip closure, 55
infants, 188–189

L
Listerine,
    ingredients in, 174
    litmus paper, 56–57, 135

M
minerals,
    calcium fluorapatite, 47
    calcium hydroxyapatite, 46–47
mixed dentition, 120
moderate fluorosis, 102
money and ethics, clashed, 21
mouth chemistry,
    acidity, control, 37
    affected by, 35
    circumstances, elevating risk of
        developing cavities, 36–37
    dry mouth, side effect of, 35
    life situations, influence, 36
    saliva, *see* saliva
    women, during pregnancy, 36

N
National Call to Action, General Richard
    H. Carmona's document, 26
new techniques in dentistry,
    DIAGNOdent laser, 15
    Digital Imaging Fiber-Optic Trans-
        Illumination, 15
    InspektorPro, 15

O
odontoblasts, 116
Opalescence, 120
oral health in America, 25

P
paranoid tooth flossers, 163
periodontal treatment, 72
periodontitis, 78–79
pH measurement, 56
plaque, linked with, 67
prenatal care, 188
preteens and teens, 195–198

preventive dental program, 22
preventive dentistry, 23, 25
prophylactic squads, 24

R
rebuilding teeth, believe in, 11
remineralization, meaning of, 48
    fluoride, role of, 48
    xylitol, role of, 48
root resorption, 117

S
saliva,
    acidic or alkaline, 54
    acidity, changes in, 36, 53
    aging, 63–64
    amount of, 55
    benefits of, 54
    esophagus, protection, 27
    flows, measured by, 55
    medication, side effects of, 63
    test, 57–59
sealants,
    alternative ways, 112
    bacteria, blocked by, 109
    children, for, 110
    meaning of, 107–108
    xylitol, comparison with, 111
senile dementia, 91
silver filling, 12
    mercury, releasing from, 124
    pros and cons of, 12–14
sodium fluoride, 96–97, 99, 103, 173, 175, 198
stannous fluoride, 96–97
sticky spots, 9
strong teeth, 45

T
teeth, sensitivity, 49
toddlers, 191–194
toothbrushing, 168-171
tooth damage, cause of, 4
tooth decay, epidemic of, 22

tooth-corrosive acids, 41
tooth-protective food, 22, 62, 133, 138
V
Vipeholm study, 42–43

W
white spot lesions, 71
whitening, demand for, 113

X
xylitol,
    acceptance among dental
        professionals, 154–156
    alkalizing benefits, 148
    benefits of eating, 149
    birch trees, extracted from, 145
    calcium, benefit on absorption of, 148
    cavity prevention, 151–152
    cavity-forming bacteria, remove, 146
    diabetic sugar, used as, 156
    dose of, 148
    ear infections, 150
    early cavities, repair, 152–153
    early history of, 146–147
    harmful bacteria, unable to use, 149
    laxative effect, 157
    meals, after, 157–158
    natural healing process, stimulates, 149
    pets, not given to, 157
    proponent of, 4
    questions, 203–205
    recent studies, 147–149
    sources of, 145
    sugar alcohol, different from, 157
    treatments, reduce, 158
    ways to eat, 156–157
xylose, 148

Y
young children, 194–195
Z
Zellies, 147, 194
Zellies toothbrush, 169

Made in the USA
Coppell, TX
11 February 2020